GeoJournal Library

Volume 126

More information about this series at http://www.springer.com/series/6007

Kim M. Lersch · Jayajit Chakraborty
Editors

Geographies of Behavioural Health, Crime, and Disorder

The Intersection of Social Problems and Place

Springer

Editors
Kim M. Lersch
School of Information
University of South Florida
Tampa, FL, USA

Jayajit Chakraborty
Department of Sociology and Anthropology
The University of Texas at El Paso
El Paso, TX, USA

ISSN 0924-5499 ISSN 2215-0072 (electronic)
GeoJournal Library
ISBN 978-3-030-33466-6 ISBN 978-3-030-33467-3 (eBook)
https://doi.org/10.1007/978-3-030-33467-3

This Springer imprint is published by the registered company Springer Nature Switzerland AG
The registered company address is: Gewerbestrasse 11, 6330 Cham, Switzerland

Contents

Chapter 1
Introduction: Connecting Behavioral Health, Crime, and Neighborhood Disorder

Kim M. Lersch and Jayajit Chakraborty

The impetus for this edited volume began after attending a symposium titled "Falling through the Cracks[1]" that examined the intersection between the mental health and the criminal justice systems. The panel of speakers addressed a number of critical issues pertaining to the status of mental health care in the United States, including access to treatment for substance abuse and behavioral health disorders; the role of jails and prisons in containing the mentally ill; and the general public's fear of those with a mental illness. This trepidation often leads to calls for service to the police to control the 'problem,' whether it be complaints of homelessness; panhandling; disturbing the peace; or, in some cases, valid concerns regarding the behavior of a violent person struggling with their disorder. Serving in their peace-keeping role, law enforcement officers are often transformed into "street-corner psychiatrists" and act as gatekeepers for both the criminal justice and mental health care systems (Teplin 2000).

Essentially, the police have three options when dealing with individuals with mental illness. First, the officer may make an arrest and transport the individual to jail. Estimates of the rates of persons with a mental illness in local jails vary widely, from a low of 6% to as many as 64% of jail detainees reporting some sort of mental disorder (Morabito and Wilson 2017). The National Alliance on Mental

[1]Falling through the Cracks: The Intersection between the Mental Health and Criminal Justice Systems. University of South Florida, College of Behavioral & Community Sciences, October 6, 2017.

K. M. Lersch (✉)
School of Information, University of South Florida, Tampa, FL, USA
e-mail: klersch@usf.edu

J. Chakraborty
Department of Sociology and Anthropology, The University of Texas at El Paso, El Paso, TX, USA
e-mail: jchakraborty@utep.edu

K. M. Lersch and J. Chakraborty (eds.), *Geographies of Behavioural Health, Crime, and Disorder*, GeoJournal Library 126,
https://doi.org/10.1007/978-3-030-33467-3_1

Illness (n.d.) estimates that approximately 15% of men and 30% of women in jails have a serious mental disorder. The problem is that jails simply are not equipped to properly care for persons with a mental illness. A recent report (AbuDagga et al. 2016) found that one-third of jails reported that despite the fact that the staff had limited training, a substantial amount of time and effort was focused on caring for individuals with serious mental health disorders. Further, incarcerated individuals with a mental illness are more likely to be charged with rule violations within the correctional setting and are at greater risk for assaults, both as the victim and as the perpetrator (Bronson and Berzofsky 2017; DeHart and Iachini 2019; James and Glaze 2006).

A second option available to law enforcement officers is to initiate an involuntary civil commitment (IC) to a mental health facility. The exact criteria for this process may vary based on jurisdiction (Sheehan 2009). In the U.S., most states require the presence of dangerousness in order to initiate compulsory confinement. That is, a person must pose an imminent threat to either self (suicide) or others (homicide) in order to be taken into custody (Testa and West 2010). The problem with this rather stringent standard is that there are individuals with serious mental health disorders that are not dangerous but still refuse medical treatment. If there is no threat of immediate danger, the person cannot be forced into hospitalization even though a clear need for intervention and treatment is present.

This leaves the police with their third option: "informal dispositions," or essentially, do their best to calm the person without taking any formal action. As discussed by Teplin (2000) this is normally the first choice of police officers on the scene. Teplin stated that "Officers' decisions to hospitalize, arrest, or deal with a mentally ill person informally are based less on the degree of symptomatology than on the demands and constraints of the situation (p. 10)." Police officers modify their behavior based on the sociodemographic characteristics of the community, citizen demands for service, and workload. In some areas, officers may be actively discouraged from taking formal actions with the mentally ill because of system overload: There simply is no place to take non-violent individuals (Lersch 2018).

Kim Lersch had the opportunity to observe the rather dramatic difference that geography can make on the actions of law enforcement officers. While working on a Federally funded research project to assess substance abuse among arrestees at two jails in neighboring counties in the state of Florida, the primary charges for detainees varied greatly depending on the county. The first county was known for tourism and covered a relatively small area. It was very common for the research team to see a relatively steady stream of arrestees for minor offenses that are often associated with mental illness: intoxication; minor drug possession; trespassing; public urination; vagrancy; and disturbing the peace. The terms of the grant required the hiring of several correctional officers to assist the team. As there was little to no overtime available to the detention deputies, there were no issues with finding individuals who were interested in working on the project.

The second jail was less than 30 miles from the first location, but the two facilities were worlds apart. Because the detention deputies were already working as much overtime as their contract allowed, only supervisory staff could be hired to assist the research team. The primary charges for the arrestees were for serious criminal offenses only; one simply did not see individuals brought to the jail for non-violent, quality of life offenses. The difference was so striking that one of the supervisors was asked about the issue. He indicated that law enforcement officers were strongly discouraged from bringing in offenders unless the charge was serious due to the overcrowded conditions at the jail.

So, what happens to those suffering from mental illness in these two counties? Because of the high arrest rate for non-violent offenses in the first county, it is possible for an individual to have multiple arrests and convictions for the same misdemeanor offense. Depending on the nature of the charge/conviction, after multiple convictions for the same crime the charge may be elevated to a felony. Conviction for a felony may result in sentencing to prison and, if the individual has a long list of misdemeanor convictions, the term of confinement may be longer.

In the second county, one can safely assume that while arrests are not often made, relatively minor offenses still occur. Because individuals are not taken into custody, the actions of the non-violent mentally ill are not criminalized. But do these individuals receive any sort of treatment for their disorders? And how did the criminal justice system become so involved with the mentally ill? While a number of explanations have been proffered, two factors are consistently in the discussion: the deinstitutionalization movement and the media portrayal of the mentally ill as violent, demonized individuals.

The deinstitutionalization movement began in the post-World War II era as a response to growing concern over the confinement of mentally ill persons in large state institutions, often in less than ideal conditions. Prior to this time, the institutionalization of the mentally ill was seen as beneficial and therapeutic. This philosophy of confinement reached its peak level in 1955, when nearly half a million patients were housed in state institutions. A number of contributory factors led to dramatic changes in the care and treatment of those diagnosed with mental illness, including growing scrutiny, medical advances, and economic incentives.

As argued by Bassuk and Gerson (1978), the public became more concerned with the prevalence, treatment, and prevention of mental disorders when large numbers of recruits were rejected from military service due to serious psychiatric disorders. This new realization of the plight of the mentally ill led to an increase in funding for research and training to improve the delivery of services. The growing awareness of mistreatment, abuse, and inhumane conditions that existed in many of the state institutions became a driving force for change not only for the public, but for the medical and psychiatric communities as well.

Advances in medical treatment led to the development of antipsychotic drugs including Thorazine and phenothiazine, which made it possible to control the symptoms of psychosis, including hallucinations, delusions, depression, and anxiety (Bassuk and Gerson 1978; Kim 2016; Raphael and Stoll 2013; Fuller Torrey 2015). This was a new revelation in the care of the mentally ill, as inpatient hospitalization was no longer required for individuals suffering from this condition. This discovery fueled the growing belief among health professionals that mental illnesses could be cured. As the use of antipsychotic drugs became more widespread, larger numbers of individuals were released from institutions. The demand for community-based treatment programs was growing.

Finally, a number of changes in the economic funding for the management of mental illness were driven by the Community Mental Health Act of 1963. This legislation provided federal funding to the states for the development of community mental health centers, which would replace the need for large in-patient state hospitals in caring for those with chronic mental illnesses. As an added financial incentive, a number of federal initiatives such as Supplemental Security Income (SSI), Social Security Disability Insurance (SSDI), Medicaid, Medicare, food stamps, and other programs provided financial support for mentally ill individuals who were living in the community. If a mentally ill person was living in a state-run facility, then s/he was not eligible for these federal assistance programs. Since the state-run facilities were funded almost exclusively with state dollars, it was fiscally beneficial for states to discharge patients and take advantage of the federal support for this population (Kim 2016; Fuller Torrey 2015). Thus, the deinstitutionalization movement was born, leading to a 95% drop in the population held in state mental institutions over a fifty-year period (Fisher et al. 2009; Schutt 2016; Swanson 2015).

Unfortunately, the promise of effective community-based mental health care was never realized. Insufficient funding, lack of adequate systems to administer and monitor follow-up care, and the use of unproven therapeutic techniques led to what has been described as a "non-system of community aftercare (Bassuk and Gerson 1978: 48)." Fuller Torrey (2015) argues that there are currently more than 1 million individuals in the U.S. living in the community who would have previously been institutionalized in the 1950s. Additionally, Torrey estimates that there are at least 3.2 million people diagnosed with serious mental illnesses living in our neighborhoods that are not receiving treatment for their conditions. This figure is based on statistics released by the National Institute of Mental Health, which indicate that 40% of adults with schizophrenia and 51% of adults with severe bipolar disorder receive no treatment in any given year.

Coinciding with the deinstitutionalization movement was a sharp increase in the number of incarcerated individuals in the U.S. A number of researchers have attributed the increase in the prison population to deinstitutionalization (Swanson 2015; Raphael and Stoll 2013). This follows the "Penrose Hypothesis," first argued by Lionel Penrose in 1939. In an analysis of European incarceration and institutionalization rates, Penrose found an inverse relationship between the populations of mental health institutions and prisons. This led Penrose to conclude that if one form of confinement is increased, the other will decrease (Lamb 2015; Penrose 1939). While Penrose came to this conclusion decades before deinstitutionalization began, the merits of his premise continue to be argued in contemporary times. A recent survey by the Treatment Advocacy Center reported that in the majority of states, the largest prison or jail confined more individuals with a serious mental illness than the largest state hospital (Swanson 2015). As stated by Kim (2016: 10), "In sum, as a result of deinstitutionalization, the mentally ill who would have been previously institutionalized in mental hospitals are at risk of being homeless, involved in crime, subject to arrest, and finally held up in jails and prisons due to a lack of personal and community resources."

Thus far, this introduction has focused on the relationship between mental health and arrests for relatively minor, social disorder offenses. This is much more common than arrests for violent behavior. However, this differs from the picture that is portrayed in the media, where individuals with serious mental illnesses are painted as violent, dangerous, and unpredictable. This is especially true given a number of highly publicized mass shootings that occurred over the past decade and the resulting political debate surrounding gun ownership among those diagnosed with a serious mental illness. The Sandy Hook shooting in 2012 in which Adam Lanza shot and killed 20 children and 5 adults; the Aurora, Colorado movie theatre mass shooting incident by James Holmes in which a dozen were killed and another 70 injured; Jared Loughner's actions at a political rally in which U.S. Congresswoman Gabrielle Giffords and 6 others were shot; and most recently the incident in Parkland, Florida, when gunman Nikolas Crus killed 17 students and staff members at a high school: All of these incidents have all fueled the public's fear of the mentally ill (Metzl and MacLeish 2015). As argued by Knoll and Annas (2016), initial media coverage of a mass shooting may label the shooter as "mentally unstable" or "mentally ill" even before any definitive facts have been unearthed. The result is that the mentally ill face greater stigmitization and apprehension than ever before, even though a causal link between mental illness, violence, and mass shootings has not been supported by the evidence (Wilson et al. 2016; Wahl 2003).

According to surveys, the mass media are the most common sources of public information about mental illness (Wahl 2003). Unfortunately, content analyses consistently find that stories of mental illness are dominated by themes of dangerousness, unpredictability, and violence (see, for example, Day and Page 1986; Philo et al. 1999; Wahl et al. 2002). Further, the portrayal of the mentally ill in fictional and non-fictional crime-based television programs tends to confirm negative stereotypes (Parrott and Parrott 2015). These constant negative images of the mentally ill can have a strong impact on public opinion, which can result in acts of discrimination in employment, housing, health care, and social gatherings (Parrott and Parrott 2015; Wahl 2003). Those suffering from a mental illness may also be discouraged from seeking help, fearing the impact of being labeled and stereotyped solely by their disorder (Corrigan 2004).

We echo the conclusions reached at the symposium attended so many months ago: issues related to behavioral health, crime, and disorder are inextricably linked. In this collection of interdisciplinary and original works, a variety of contemporary topics related to the importance of place on the quality of community health and well-being are examined. Each chapter introduces the reader to an overview of the topic, presents theoretical frameworks and the latest empirical evidence, and discusses real world policy implications and solutions. Focusing on some of the most critical contemporary social problems, including the opioid crisis, suicide, crime, homelessness, and social and environmental justice, each unique contribution discusses the importance of geography in our quality of life.

In Chap. 2, Lersch and Christy explore the geographic distribution of mental health-related 911 calls for service in the City of Detroit, Michigan. Statistically significant hot and cold spots were identified for various categories of mental health calls, including suicides and suicide attempts as well as people with mental illness who were reported to be violent and non-violent. Additionally, various characteristics of the physical/built environment were examined to see if there was a relationship between place and mental health related calls for service. While the locations of crimes of violence do influence risk of calls for service for mental health issues, locations of non-violent property crimes, blight violations, and quality of life offenses were found to have a greater influence on the risk of suicide, non-violent mental health, and violent mental health calls for service.

In Chap. 3, Vaughan presents an overview of the opioid crisis, focusing on the various approaches used to measure the level of community involvement. In the U. S., many researchers and policy makers focus on the metric of overdose deaths associated with opioids as the benchmark for assessing the importance of the crisis in a given area. As argued by Vaughan, death tells but one side of the story, and using this single measure may seriously underestimate the true level of involvement. Vaughan presents the many ways of measuring the opioid crisis in order to provide a better foundation for comparisons across different jurisdictions and eventually developing policy that is congruent with the needs of the community.

In Chap. 4, Hart presents an overview of some of the most commonly used methods to identify crime "hot spots." Understanding where and when crime and disorder cluster, both spatially and temporally, provides vital information necessary for community leaders to design and implement effective crime-reduction strategies and community-safety initiatives. These techniques generally fall into three different categories: retrospective; prospective; and predictive policing analytics. Until recently researchers and analysts have operated *retrospectively*—using incident location information to describe historical crime patterns through the use of data visualization techniques or to design reactionary policing strategies based on the assumption that historical crime patterns are reliable indicators of future problem areas. Predictive analytical techniques are the next generation of crime analysis and intelligence-led policing, in which patterns in crime data are exploited dynamically and prevent crime through *proactive* allocation of resources.

In Chap. 5, Brantingham et al. review methodologies used to identify, analyze, and predict spatial and temporal concentrations of crime and disorder. Analysis of crime hot spots (spatial concentrations) and burning times (temporal concentrations) have become a major component of the work of criminologists, crime analysts, and crime prevention practitioners. This chapter discusses the strengths and weaknesses of several traditional and contemporary hot spot analysis methods, as well as relevant theoretical frameworks. A key contribution is an expanded theoretical model for crime hot spot formation, grounded in crime pattern theory, which provides an improved understanding of how such hot spots are created and has important implications for crime hot spot prevention and related policies.

In Chap. 6, Lynch et al. focus on assessing the geographic distribution of green/environmental crimes and its social determinants across U.S. states. Although issues of environmental crime and victimization have received increased attention in recent years, the authors emphasize that traditional criminological questions and methodologies have not been extensively applied to studying geographies of green crime. Using the U.S. EPA's Environmental Compliance History data, they construct state-level indicators of environmental crimes and compare them to corresponding measures of street crime. Their study also examines how welfare expenditures and racial/ethnic composition of states also influence the geographic distribution of environmental crimes.

In Chap. 7, Chataway and Bourke provide a detailed review of emerging scholarship on an interdisciplinary topic: fear of crime and disorder. This chapter discusses how fear of crime and disorderly environments can impact an individual's quality of life and physical wellbeing, as well as the broader implications that fear of crime may have on the functioning of society. The authors introduce a working definition of fear of crime that considers this issue as a social-psychological process. They also review the common methods used to evaluate fear of crime and perceptions of neighborhood disorder, as well as individual, neighborhood, and societal level factors influencing fear of crime. The authors conclude that common predictors of fear of crime could be better converged using contemporary social-psychological models that consider the interactions between vulnerability/risk perceptions, perceptions of social and physical environment, and worry about crime.

In Chap. 8, Oudshoorn focuses on a particular type of social disorder: homelessness, which is explored here as a fusion policy problem. The author argues that homelessness is a policy problem because the structure of social systems creates risk for housing loss and determines supports available in the case of homelessness, and a fusion policy problem due to several related but often disconnected systems such as health care, justice, housing, income support, violence against women/family violence services, and other social services. Homeless individuals pose special challenges for communities especially if mental health treatment is necessary. This chapter provides a detailed overview of factors and policies that cause homelessness, and explores several areas of potential policy intervention for homelessness prevention.

In Chap. 9, Nadybal et al. provide an interdisciplinary and international perspective on environmental justice (EJ) activism, research, and policy. Over the last few decades, EJ has evolved into both a body of academic scholarship and a social movement that seeks to identify, document, and address environmental discrimination and related injustices faced by various socially disadvantaged population groups. This chapter discusses theoretical foundations of EJ and related concepts, findings from EJ-oriented studies in the US and elsewhere, new fields relying on EJ methodologies, and both the global and local implications of achieving EJ. While no single chapter can fully summarize the entire EJ research literature, this chapter provides a comprehensive overview that emphasizes the importance of EJ in restoring justice and equity for those who need it most.

We sincerely hope that readers will enjoy these outstanding contributions from our diverse body of scholars. Without their efforts, this collection would not have been possible.

References

AbuDagga, A., Wolfe, S., Carome, M., Phatdouang, A., & Torrey, E. (2016). *Individuals with serious mental illnesses in county jails: A survey of jail staff's perspectives*. Washington, DC: Public Citizen's Health Research Group & The Treatment Advocacy Center.

Bassuk, E. L., & Gerson, S. (1978). Deinstitutionalization and mental health services. *AMHC Forum, 31*(2), 39–46. Retrieved from https://www.ncbi.nlm.nih.gov/pubmed/10297338.

Bronson, J., & Berzofsky, M. (2017). *Indicators of mental health problems reported by prisoners and jail inmates, 2011–12*. Bureau of Justice Statistics: Special Report. Washington, DC: United States Department of Justice.

Corrigan, P. (2004). How stigma interferes with mental health care. *American Psychologist, 59,* 614–625.

Day, D. M., & Page, S. (1986). Portrayal of mental illness in Canadian newspapers. *Canadian Journal of Psychiatry, 31,* 813–816.

DeHart, D., & Iachini, A. L. (2019). Mental health & trauma among incarcerated persons: Development of a training curriculum for correction officers. *American Journal of Criminal Justice, 44,* 457–473.

Fisher, W. H., Geller, J. L., & Pandiani, J. A. (2009). The changing role of the state psychiatric hospital. *Health Affairs, 28*(3). Available online at https://doi.org/10.1377/hlthaff.28.3.676. Accessed July 1, 2019.

Fuller Torrey, E. (2015). Deinstitutionalization and the rise of violence. *CNS Spectrums, 20*(3), 207–214. https://doi.org/10.1017/S1092852914000753.

James, D., & Glaze, L. (2006). *Mental health problems of prison and jail inmates. Bureau of Justice Statistics Special Report*. Washington, DC: United States Department of Justice.

Knoll, J. L., IV., & Annas, G. D. (2016). *Mass shootings and mental illness.* Available at https://www.psychiatryonline.org/doi/pdf/10.5555/appi.books.9781615371099.

Kim, D. (2016). Psychiatric deinstitutionalization and prison population growth. *Criminal Justice Policy Review, 27*(1), 3–21. https://doi.org/10.1177/0887403414547043.

Lamb, R. H. (2015). Does institutionalization cause criminalization? The Penrose hypothesis. *JAMA Psychiatry, 72*(2), 105–106.

Lersch, K. M. (2018). Policing urban spaces. In C. Crawford & R. Burns (Eds.), *Spatial policing: The influence of time, space, and geography on law enforcement practices*. Durham: Carolina Academic Press.

Metzl, J. M., & MacLeish, K. T. (2015). Mental illness, mass shootings, and the politics of American Firearms. *American Journal of Public Health, 105*(2), 240–249.

Morabito, M. S., & Wilson, A. B. (2017). Selecting a method of case identification to estimate the involvement of people with mental illnesses in the criminal justice system: A research note. *International Journal of Offender Therapy and Comparative Criminology, 61*(8), 919–937. https://doi.org/10.1177/0306624X15608823.

National Alliance on Mental Illness. (n.d.). *Jailing people with mental illness*. https://www.nami.org/Learn-More/Public-Policy/Jailing-People-with-Mental-Illness. Accessed June 25, 2019.

Parrott, S., & Parrott, C. T. (2015). Law & disorder: The portrayal of mental illness in U.S. crime dramas. *Journal of Broadcasting & Electronic Media, 59*(4), 640–657.

Penrose, L. S. (1939). Mental disease and crime: Outline of a comparative study of European statistics. *British Journal of Medical Psychology, 18*(1), 1–15. https://doi.org/10.1111/j.2044-8341.1939.tb00704.x.

Philo, G., Secker, J., Platt, S., Henderson, L., McLaughlin, G., & Burnside, J. (1999). The impact of the mass media on public images of mental illness: Media content and audience belief. *Health Education Journal, 53,* 271–281.

Raphael, S., & Stoll, M. A. (2013). Assessing the contribution of the deinstitutionalization of the mentally ill to growth in the U.S. incarceration rate. *The Journal of Legal Studies, 42*(1), 187–222. https://doi.org/10.1086/667773.

Schutt, R. K. (2016). *Social environment and mental illness: The progress and paradox of deinstitutionalization. 50 years after deinstitutionalization: Mental illness in contemporary communities* (pp. 91–118). Emerald Group Publishing Limited. https://doi.org/10.1108/S1057-629020160000017004.

Sheehan, K. (2009). Compulsory treatment in psychiatry. *Current Opinion in Psychiatry, 22*(6), 582–586.

Swanson, S. (2015, April 30). *A shocking number of mentally ill Americans end up in prison instead of treatment.* Washingtonpost.Com.

Teplin, L. A. (2000). Keeping the peace: Police discretion and mentally ill persons. *National Institute of Justice Journal, 244,* 8–15.

Testa, M., & West, S. G. (2010). Civil commitment in the United States. *Psychiatry (Edgmont), 7* (10), 30–40.

Wahl, O. F. (2003). News media portrayal of mental illness. *American Behavioral Scientist, 46* (12), 1594–1600. https://doi.org/10.1177/0002764203254615.

Wahl, O. F., Wood, A., & Richards, R. (2002). Newspaper coverage of mental illness: Is it changing? *Psychiatric Rehabilitation Skills, 6,* 9–31.

Wilson, L. C., Ballman, A. D., & Buczek, T. J. (2016). News content about mass shootings and attitudes toward mental illness. *Journalism & Mass Communication Quarterly, 93*(3), 644–658. https://doi.org/10.1177/1077699015610064.

Part I
Geography and Behavioral Health

Chapter 2
The Geography of Mental Health: An Examination of Police Calls for Service

Kim M. Lersch and Annette Christy

2.1 Introduction

Mental illnesses are one of the most common health conditions in the United States (Centers for Disease Control and Prevention 2018b). One in five adults, approximately 43.4 million adults in 2015, had any mental illness in the previous year (Bose et al. 2016). An estimated 9.8 million adults (1 in 25) were identified as having a "serious mental illness," which is defined as a "mental, behavioral, or emotional disorder resulting in serious functional impairment, which substantially interferes with or limits one or more major life activities" (National Institute of Mental Health 2019).

The impacts of mental illness may be experienced not only by the individual diagnosed with the disorder, but by his or her family members, the community, and a variety of public resources, such as physicians, hospitals, police departments, correctional facilities, and the criminal justice system. There were nearly 66 million visits in 2014 to physicians with mental health disorders as the primary diagnosis (CDC 2018a). Mood disorders for young people and adults age 18–44 are one of the most common causes for hospitalization. Furthermore, it has been estimated that the total cost of lost earnings due to serious mental health issues are greater than $193 billion per year.

It is not uncommon for people with a mental illness to interaction with law enforcement, either in the form of an arrest or a call for service (Livingston 2016; Yang et al. 2018) although the reported rates vary widely. In a review of relevant studies, Livingston found that 1 in 4 persons diagnosed with a mental illness had

K. M. Lersch (✉)
School of Information, University of South Florida, Tampa, USA
e-mail: klersch@usf.edu

A. Christy
Department of Mental Health, Law, & Policy, University of South Florida, Tampa, USA
e-mail: achristy@usf.edu

K. M. Lersch and J. Chakraborty (eds.), *Geographies of Behavioural Health, Crime, and Disorder*, GeoJournal Library 126,
https://doi.org/10.1007/978-3-030-33467-3_2

been arrested at some point in their lives. Rates of police calls related to mental illness vary from as low as 1% to as high as 49% (Livingston 2016; Wilson-Bates 2008). The strain on police resources can be especially acute in rural areas, where police may be seen as the only viable resource for those seeking assistance for individuals with mental disorders (Weisheit et al. 2006; Yang et al. 2018).

Relatively few studies have focused on the interactions of the police and people with mental illness, despite the importance of the issue. While some work examining the spatial-temporal concentrations of police calls for service with persons diagnosed with serious mental health issues exists, little has been done to understand these patterns (Vaughan et al. 2018b). The present study seeks to address this gap.

The purpose of this chapter is to explore the geographic distribution of mental health-related 911 calls for service in the City of Detroit, Michigan. Using risk terrain modeling, various characteristics of the physical/built environment were examined to see if there was a relationship between place and mental health related calls for service. Specifically, the following research questions were investigated:

- Is there evidence of spatial clustering of mental health related calls for service, or are these calls randomly distributed throughout the City?
- Are there identifiable risk factors in the environment that place residents at higher risk for 911 calls related to mental health issues?
- Are there aspects of the environment that may serve as protective factors for the occurrence of emergency calls for mental health related issues?

To explore the statistical significance of the potential aggravating and protective factors, RTMDx software was used. RTMDx was developed through a grant from the U.S. Department of Justice awarded to the Rutgers Center on Public Security (see rutgerscps.org for more information).

2.2 The Geography of Mental Health

As a field of inquiry within academic geography, mental health geography is a relatively small, but growing, area of research (Philo 2005). Faris and Dunham (1939) conducted one of the first studies in the US that examined the spatial epidemiology of mental illness. Without the aid of sophisticated software, the home addresses of 34,864 people admitted to hospitals and sanitariums in Chicago from 1922 to 1934 were mapped. Definite ecological patterns were found between the rates of admissions and the structure of the city, especially with respect to schizophrenia. Overall, the rates of admissions in the more socially disorganized central areas of the city were the highest; the rates steadily decreased as one moved farther into the outskirts in the suburban areas.

Similarly, Shaw and McKay (1942) were primarily interested in the social ecology of juvenile delinquency. As part of the Chicago School, Shaw and McKay plotted the home addresses of boys who had come in contact with the various elements of the Cook County Criminal Justice system. The findings suggested a regular decrease in the level of juvenile delinquency as one moved outward from the center of the city. Shaw and McKay explored relationships between the distributions of juvenile delinquency and other social problems, including infant mortality, tuberculosis, and mental health disorders. Not surprisingly, the rates for these various measures all decreased as one moved out of the central cities. For Shaw and McKay, juvenile delinquency was just another indicator of "sickness" within a neighborhood. Other factors, such as high levels of unemployment, death, poverty, and residential turnover were also associated with socially disorganized communities.

Contemporary studies continue to advance knowledge of the relationship between neighborhood characteristics and mental health issues. Employing more and more sophisticated statistical analyses (see, for example, Chang et al. 2011; Jones 2007; Kirchner and Shiffman 2016), many researchers utilize data from the Census to measure social indicators at the tract, city, county, state, or other areal unit thought to represent neighborhoods. Social disorganization, urbanization, poverty, unemployment, lack of stable housing, level of education, and median income are frequently used sociodemographic predictors of mental illness (Rehkopf and Buka 2006; Stack 2000a, b; Trgovac et al. 2015; Vaughan et al. 2019).

It has been argued that community disorder may lead to higher levels of stress exposure, ultimately resulting in higher levels of mental illness. As argued by Turner et al. (2013, p. 258), "community disorder…presents residents with observable signs that social control is weak and that there is little concern or ability to maintain a safe and orderly physical environment. Such neighborhoods or often characterized by rundown buildings, graffiti, litter, public drinking and drug use, vandalism, and cues that crime is common." Focusing on the mental health of juveniles, Turner et al. posited that exposure to violence and victimization was an additional source of stress. When high levels of crime and victimization were combined with other forms of community disorder, the resulting stress affected mental health.

One of the weaknesses with many studies that examine the impact of neighborhood characteristics on the mental health of the individual is that the home address or zip code of the person at the time of hospitalization is often used. As argued by Helbich (2017), this practice is problematic on several levels. For illustrative purposes, let us envision a hypothetical individual, Joe, who has recently been hospitalized for depression and suicidal ideations. Joe's home address is located within a specific census tract. While this administrative unit is useful for researchers, the boundaries do not coincide with the area Joe views as "his" neighborhood. Joe becomes a statistic, where his individual status is now defined by aggregated characteristics of a neighborhood that does not exist.

Furthermore, the fluidity of movement through time and space is ignored when Joe's area of spatial influence is reduced to a single address—his home. Exposures to other environments as Joe conducts the routine activities of his life (i.e., going to work, school, entertainment centers, etc.) are ignored. Helbich (2018b) pointed out that 80% of the daily activity space of individuals is outside of the area perceived to be their home neighborhood. While Joe's neighborhood may be marked by high levels of disorder, crime, and other stressors, as he travels to his work place Joe may walk through areas that have much higher levels of social cohesion and positive environmental factors that may in turn have a stabilizing impact on his emotional health. Due to these limitations, there is a growing body of research that puts greater emphasis on movement through time and space, attempting to measure the dynamic impact of environmental exposures on the mental health of individuals (Drawve et al. 2015; Helbich 2018a, b; Kirchner and Shiffman 2016; Philo 2005; Vaughan et al. 2018a, b). Street network patterns, activity nodes and pathways, and other aspects of the physical and built environment at the micro level become critical components in the examination of risk and protective factors for stressors, crime, and overall quality of life.

2.3 The Special Case of Suicide

Suicide is the 10th leading cause of death in the U.S., and the rate has been rising over the past decade (CDC 2018b). Interestingly, in a study of 2015 data from the National Violent Death Reporting System, CDC researchers found that more than half of the individuals who died by suicide had no known diagnosed mental health condition at the time of their death. This makes prevention efforts difficult, as there is no "easy" way to identify and support people at risk of suicide. Even among those who have attempted suicide, ultimately the majority do not move on to a completed suicide (Hempstead 2006).

Similar to the study of the geography of mental illness, a number of researchers have examined the spatial concentration of suicides (Trgovac et al. 2015), Many studies have focused on the level of social integration and regulation in communities (Trgovac et al. 2015) Common predictors of social integration and regulation include rural versus urban environments, economic factors, housing stability, marital status, and religiosity (Recker and Moore 2016). Much of this research was driven by Durkheim's classic theory of suicide, which argued that suicide and other social pathologies are driven by the structure of social relationships (Abrutyn and Mueller 2014; Durkheim 1857/1951; Recker and Moore 2016).

2.4 Purpose of the Present Study

The present study focused on the geographic patterns of mental health related calls for service to the police. Rather than focusing on the home address of the individual in crisis, calls for service may occur anywhere within the landscape of the city—public spaces, streets, workplaces, etc.—essentially, any location within the activity space of the individual. Risk terrain modeling was used to analyze potential risk and protective factors in the urban landscape. Understanding these factors may assist in our understanding of why mental health issues are occurring in specific locations.

2.5 Risk Terrain Modeling

Risk Terrain Modeling (RTM) is a relatively new analytical technique developed by Caplan and Kennedy (2010) as they studied the locations of shootings in Irvington, New Jersey. Using geographic information systems (GIS) technology, spatial relationships were examined between the locations of shootings and other factors identified as potentially "risky" for the occurrence of shootings: known gang members' addresses; the locations of drug arrests; and high-risk infrastructure, which was defined as the locations of liquor stores, bars, strip clubs and fast food restaurants. The authors then employed these risk factors to develop maps to assist law enforcement personnel in the prediction of the locations of future shooting incidents, develop plans for intervention, and assess the effectiveness of the response (Caplan and Kennedy 2010, 2016).

The underlying theoretical basis for RTM is based on the notion that crime is not randomly distributed through time and place: Some locations are "riskier" than others for various forms of victimization. RTM is heavily influenced by environmental criminologists who have focused on the geography of crime, including early Chicago School theorists, routine activities and opportunity theory, and the Brantinghams' notion of environmental backcloth, crime generators, attractors, and protective factors (for a full discussion of the principles of environmental criminology, please see Brantingham et al., this volume; Hart and Lersch 2015 or Wortley and Mazerolle 2008).

On a more mechanical level, the general idea behind RTM is to create a grid of cells (say, a 500 by 500 ft raster grid) that covers the entire study area. To measure the influence of proximity, for each factor of interest a value of 1 is assigned to cells in which the risk is present (such as the area one block around a bar) while a 0 is assigned to a cell where the risk is not present (i.e., no bar is present). A risk layer can also be created the measures the influence of density, such as an entertainment area with a high concentration of bars and restaurants. An individual risk layer is created for each factor in the analysis. The different risk layers are ultimately combined into a final Risk Terrain Map in which the cell values for each corresponding 500 $\times$ 500 area are summed together (for more information on RTM, see Hart, this volume).

2.6 Study Area: The City of Detroit

The City of Detroit is located within Wayne County in Southeastern Michigan. The estimated population in 2017 was 679,865 persons (CDC 2019). The median household income was $27,838 and 37.9% of the City's residents lived in poverty (CDC 2019). The majority of residents were Black or African American (79.2%), with 14.1% White, and the remaining classified as other. The majority of Detroit residents were not Hispanic or Latino (92.4%).

There are a number of characteristics of the City of Detroit that make it unique. First and foremost is the catastrophic reduction in population. The population of the City dropped from nearly two million residents in 1950 to its current level of under 700,000 residents (Binelli 2013). A number of reasons have been given for the decline. Describing Detroit as "one of the most notorious examples of severe decline in North America," Xie et al. (2018, p. 350) noted the impact of urban sprawl, a history of racial segregation, and persistently high levels of poverty. Others (Beyer 2018; Binelli 2013) have pointed to the decline of the automotive industry, race riots, years of municipal corruption resulting in bankruptcy, poor urban planning, and high tax rates coupled with poor municipal services as key factors.

This mass exodus from the City resulted in a second unique attribute: the proliferation of abandoned and demolished structures. At the peak of the City's decline, nearly 100,000 structures stood empty and abandoned. The City encompasses an area of 139 square miles with nearly 40 square miles of vacant land due to demolitions and property abandonment (Binelli 2013).

Finally, Detroit is unique due to its consistently high crime rate. Detroit is one of the most violent cities in the world. In 2017, a total of 13,796 violent crimes were reported to the police. Every year, the Federal Bureau of Investigation (FBI) calculates crime rates for geographic areas (i.e. cities, counties, states). The violent crime rate includes murder, rape, assault, and robbery. The violent crime rate in Detroit was 2057 violent crimes per 100,000 people, which was much higher than the national level of 383 violent offenses per 100,000 (FBI 2018).

The City of Detroit completely encompasses two distinct municipalities that support their own police departments: Hamtramck and Highland Park. Comparable data were unavailable for these two cities, which were excluded from the analyses. A boundary file was downloaded from the U.S. Census Bureau for the City of Detroit. This shapefile was projected to Mercator Auxiliary Sphere with a geographic coordinate system of WGS 1984 using ArcGIS 10.6.

2.7 The Study Events, Risk Factors, and Protective Factors

The City of Detroit maintains a robust open data portal that provides access to maps and datasets focused on a variety of government services, including public safety, health, transportation, and land use (City of Detroit, n.d.). Launched in 2015, the portal was funded through a grant from the Socrata Foundation in an effort to assist in redevelopment efforts (Shueh 2015). The Open Data Portal was the source for many of the datasets used in this analysis, as can be seen in Appendix.

2.8 Dependent Variables: Mental Health Related Calls for Service

One of the datasets maintained in the Open Data Portal contains all 911 calls to the Detroit Police Department (DPD) for emergency police services and officer-initiated calls, which includes traffic stops, street stops, and observations of crimes in progress. Data collection began on September 20, 2016 and continues to the present, with data updated on a daily basis. Along with the description of the call, day, time, and other basic information, the DPD also includes latitude and longitude of the incident. To protect the identity of those involved, the DPD randomly offsets the coordinates by up to 180 ft along the street segment. From 9/20/2016 through 5/1/2019, there was a total of 28,328 calls for service that were related to mental health issues. About 1 in 7 (14.64%) of the 193,493 total calls during this time period were identified as being related to mental illness. The DPD has several different classifications that were grouped into 3 categories used in this analysis:

- Suicides (n = 8756, 4.53% of total calls): Includes call descriptions of suicide threat (n = 4985); suicide in progress (n = 3671); suicide threat or abnormal behavior (n = 47) and attempted suicide report (n = 53).
- Mental Not Violent (n = 5789, 2.99% of total calls).
- Mental Violent (n = 13,783, 7.12% of total calls): Includes call descriptions of mental violent—armed (n = 3174) and mental violent—not armed (n = 10,609).

Therefore, the analysis will explore risk factors related to (a) all mental health calls, (b) suicides, (c) not violent, persons with mental illness, (d) violent, persons with mental illness.

2.9 Potential Risk Factors

2.9.1 *Locations of Reported Crimes*

Crime locations were derived from the City of Detroit Open Data Portal using the All Crime Incidents, December 6, 2016—present file (downloaded on May 1, 2019). While a 911 call for service may or may not result in an actual reported crime, the crime incident dataset is based on information from the DPD's record management system and includes records of crimes that have been submitted to the Michigan Incident Crime Reporting and the FBI's National Incident Based Reporting System (for more information, please see Appendix). This dataset included a total of 193,493 crimes. The DPD similarly adjusted XY coordinates randomly by up to 180 ft to protect the identity of crime victims.

In addition to the more traditional classifications of property and violent crime [i.e. auto theft (n = 16,319); simple and aggravated assaults (n = 51,622); burglary (n = 18,881); homicide and attempted homicide (n = 610); larceny (n = 31,669); robbery (n = 5679); and sexual assaults (n = 1872)], a number of other criminal offenses that have been linked to overall community health and well-being were included (see Chataway and Bourke, this volume). Offense categories included sex offenses (including prostitution related offenses, n = 3448), drug offenses (n = 6288), family offenses (i.e. violent and non-violent cases of abuse, neglect, and assaults; n = 1777), and "quality of life" offenses (n = 30,845). This last category included such crimes as damage to property; disorderly conduct; gambling; liquor related offenses; obstructing the judiciary/police; and weapons related charges.

2.9.2 *Demolitions*

Through the City's Open Data portal, one can download the coordinates of residential and commercial demolitions conducted by the City or the Detroit Land Bank Authority since January 1, 2014. The data used in this analysis included 17,546 demolitions that were initiated from 1/1/2014 to 5/5/2019. This measure of demolitions does have its issues and the reader is cautioned with the interpretation of the results when it comes to this particular risk factor. Demolitions that occurred prior to 2014 are not available as the system was largely paper-based. The assumption was made that the 17,546 demolition locations were either completed and resulted in vacant lots or were uninhabited abandoned structures.

2.9.3 Blight

From September 7, 2017 through May 1, 2019, there were a total of 106,394 blight violation notices issued to property owners who violated various city ordinances that mandate minimum standards for the maintenance of commercial and residential building exteriors. These notices may be issued by city inspectors, police officers, or other city officials. While there were 242 different classifications of notices, some of the more common types included violations related to waste accumulation and disposal; inoperable vehicles; weeds and/or plant growth; graffiti; and other compliance issues. The XY coordinates for each violation were provided, along with the street address of the property where the violation occurred.

2.9.4 Businesses

When using RTM, it is common to use the locations of businesses, such as bars, restaurants, check cashing centers, automated teller machines (ATMs) or similar commercial operations as potential risk factors. These locations may provide opportunities for motivated offenders to interact with potential targets and create risky places.

When considering potential businesses that may pose greater risk for the occurrence of mental health issues, the task is a bit different from the identification of risk factors for a predatory crime such as robbery. While it makes sense to look at the potential spatial influence of convenience stores or gas stations on the risk of robbery offenses, it is more difficult to see a link between these businesses on mental health. Therefore, the potential spatial influence of two types of businesses were included in the model: licensed liquor retail outlets (which includes bars, liquor stores, restaurants, etc. that sell alcoholic beverages) and gun shops.

Liquor retail outlets were included due to the relationship between alcohol consumption and mental illness (Hartz et al. 2014; Jane-Llopis and Matytsina 2006). Problems may result from drinking too much alcohol, and some individuals may self-medicate by consuming alcoholic beverages (Mental Health Foundation 2019). There were 1026 licensed liquor outlets within the City of Detroit. These locations were found using the Open Data Portal and were geocoded based on the included latitude/longitude coordinates.

According to the Harvard School of Public Health (2019), every study that has examined the relationship between access to firearms and suicide has found a positive relationship. That is, the greater the access to firearms, the higher the suicide rate. Using Google Earth, 11 licensed gun dealers within the city limits of Detroit were identified. These locations were downloaded as a KML file and imported into the RTMDx software.

2.10 Protective Factors

Protective factors may be thought of as the opposite of a risk factor; certain aspects of the environment may reduce the risk of crime, social problems, or, in this case, mental health calls for service. For example, the area around a police department headquarters may have a lower level of crimes due to its protective nature; there may be a lower risk of victimization due to the high volume of police activity in and out of the building.

In this analysis, four factors were used to build a protective model: municipal parks (n = 338)[1]; recreational centers (n = 16); places of worship (including churches, synagogues, and mosques; n = 270); and Veterans Centers (including Veterans Administration Medical Centers, Veterans Service Centers, and Veterans Support Organizations; n = 44).

2.11 Results

The first research question explored the spatial distribution of mental health related calls for service. Specifically, are mental health related calls randomly distributed throughout the City or is there evidence of spatial clustering? To answer this question, the optimized hot spot analysis tool was used with ArcGIS 10.6. This tool uses the Getis-Ord Gi* statistic, which identifies areas where a feature has a high (or low) number of incidents and is surrounded by other features that similarly have high (or low) values (Lentz 2009). The optimized hot spot analysis tool mines the data in order to obtain parameters that will yield optimal hot spot results (Esri 2018). The tool aggregates the point data, identifies the correct scale of analysis, and automatically corrects for multiple testing and spatial dependence. Statistically significant results indicate the locations where point clusters are unusually intense or sparse.

Figure 2.1 presents the optimized hot spot analysis results for the total number of mental health related calls for service, regardless of type. The map depicts the values of the confidence level bin field. Values of either +3 or −3 are statistically significant at the 99% confidence level; +2 or −2 indicate significance at the 95% level; +1 or −1 indicate significance at the 90% level; and values of 0 indicate no significant clustering.

As can be seen in Fig. 2.1, clear hot spots and cold spots were found. Four distinct hot spot areas were found: one in the Downtown area; a second covering the neighborhoods next to the City of Highland Park; and a third the northwest neighborhoods of the city. A fourth area near in the northeastern areas near the City border with Harper Woods was also identified.

[1]While all other risk factors in this analysis were point data, the locations of the parks were in a polygon shapefile.

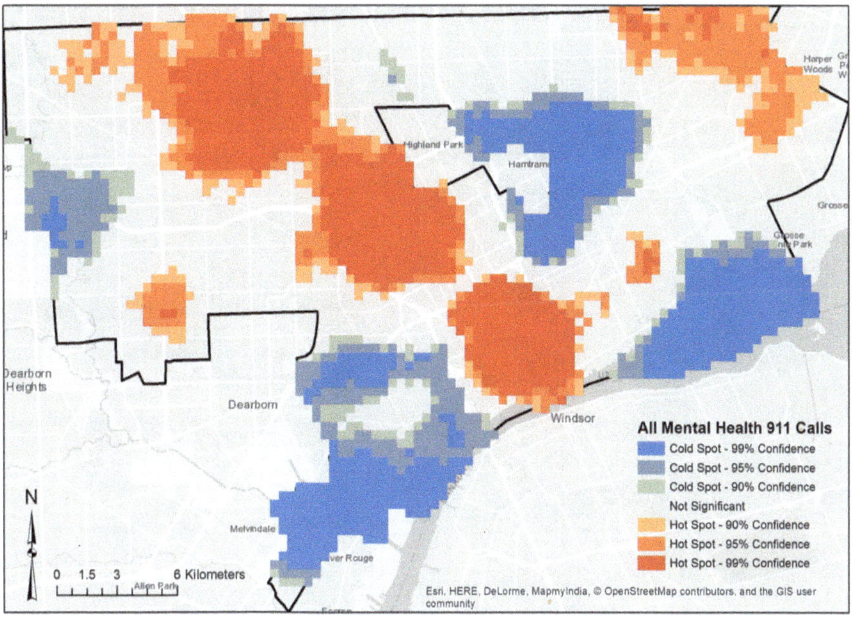

Fig. 2.1 All mental health calls for service optimized hot spot analysis

It is interesting to compare the hot and cold spot locations for the various types of mental health calls for service. As can be seen in Fig. 2.2, the locations of suicides were not randomly dispersed across the study area. Statistically significant hot and cold spots were found, and the hot spots for suicide covered smaller areas than the areas for all mental health related calls for service.

Calls for service involving persons with mental illness who were violent were also clustered in several different hot spots. The core downtown area was no longer identified as a hot spot, and there were fewer statistically significant cold spots (see Fig. 2.3).

Finally, the distribution of calls for service involving people with mental illness who were non-violent also demonstrated significant hot and cold spots. This pattern was similar to the overall distribution of mental health calls for service in the city, with the exception of the area in the northeastern part of the city. While this area had hot spots of suicides and calls for violent mentally ill persons, this area did not experience heightened levels of incidents involving people with mental illness who were non-violent (see Fig. 2.4).

The second and third research questions explored the influence of aggravating and protective factors on the level of calls for service for mental health issues. Specifically, are there identifiable factors in the environment that influence the level of risk for 911 calls related to mental health issues? To explore these questions, Risk Terrain Modeling was used to build aggravating and protective models.

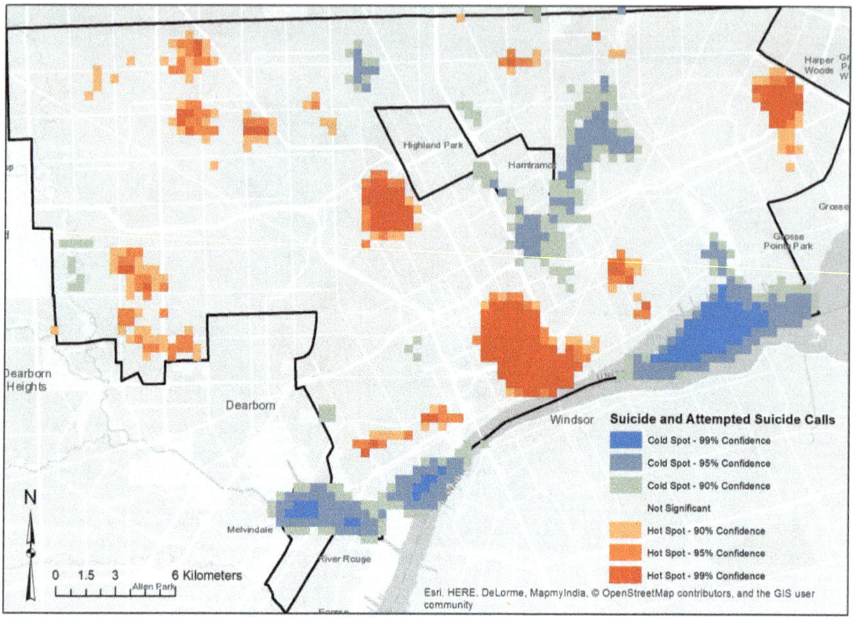

Fig. 2.2 Suicide and suicide attempts calls for service optimized hot spot analysis

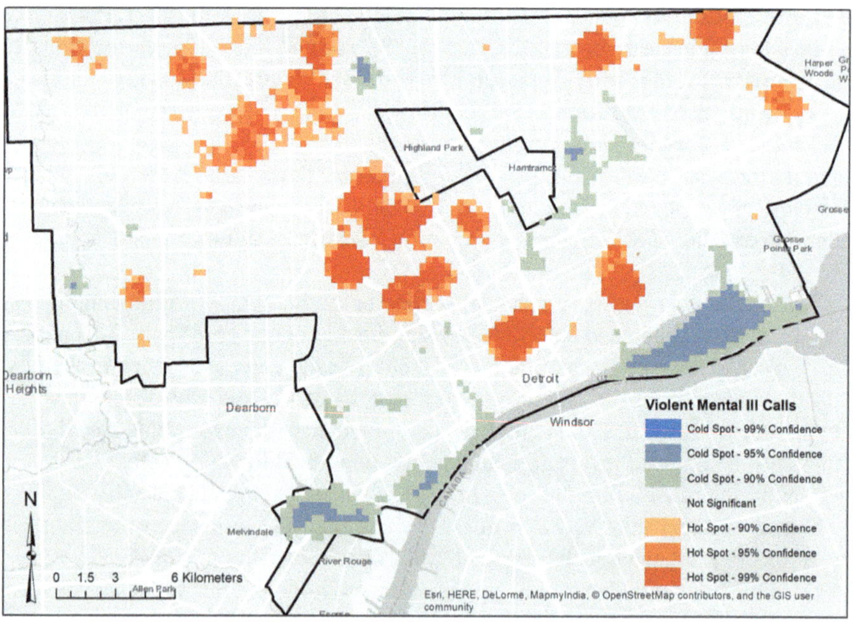

Fig. 2.3 Violent, person with mental illness: calls for service optimized hot spot analysis

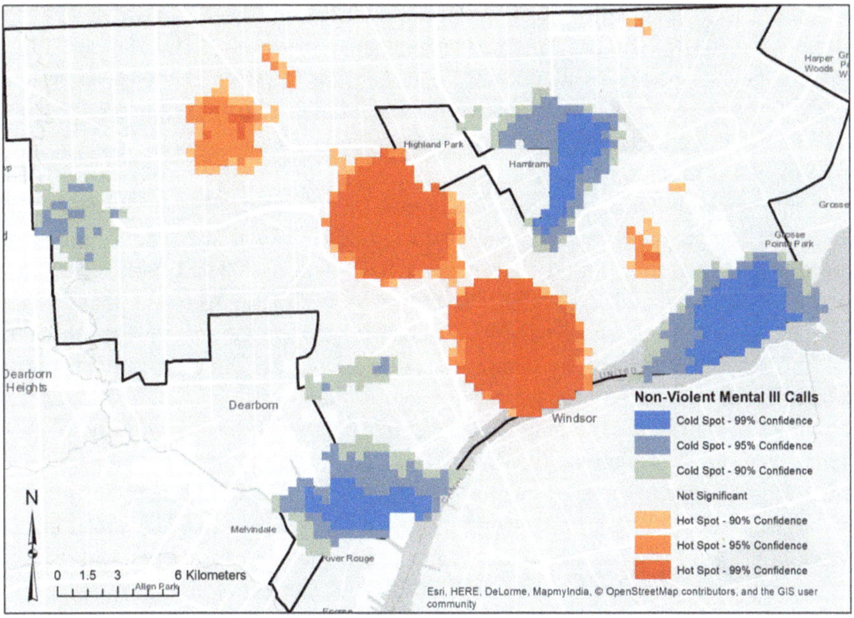

Fig. 2.4 Non-violent, person with mental illness: calls for service optimized hot spot analysis

The following risk factors were included in the analysis: assaults; blight complaints; burglaries; car theft; demolitions; drug related offenses; family offenses; gun shops; homicides and attempted homicides; larceny; liquor licenses; quality of life offenses; robbery; sex assaults; and sex offenses (see Appendix). The RTM Diagnostics software conducts tests for the spatial influence of both proximity and density of the risk factors. That is, the software tests to see if being within a specified distance from a liquor store puts one at higher risk for a mental health related incident (proximity using Euclidian distance) or if being in an area where there is a high concentration of bars and nightclubs is risky (density, as measured by kernel density). "High density" blocks are defined as those areas that are 2 standard deviations above the mean density value. The analysis unit of forecast was defined as 400 × 400 m, which resulted in a total number of 4490 places. The standard value for analysis was 800 m, which is twice the place size. Both proximity and density were tested at a distance of up to 3200 m (or 4 times the standard value size) in increments of 400 m.

The testing process began by building an elastic net penalized regression model assuming a Poisson distribution of events. Through a cross validation process, risk factors with non-zero coefficients were identified as potentially of use. These remaining variables were then used in a bidirectional step-wise regression to build a model that optimized the Bayesian Information Criteria (BIC), a score that balances the fit of the model against its complexity. The stepwise regression process was conducted for both Poisson and Negative Binomial distributions with the lowest

BIC score used to identify the appropriate distribution (for a more detailed discussion of the testing process, please see Caplan and Kennedy 2013; Heffner 2013). The coefficients in the final models are rescaled to produce relative risk values (RRVs), weighting each factor relative to one another. Finally, relative risk scores are calculated for each cell in the study area (Barnum et al. 2017).

Table 2.1 summarizes the RRVs, operationalization (either proximity or density), and spatial influence of each of the potential risk factors. If we focus attention on the risk factors for all mental health calls regardless of specific type, a number of interesting RRVs were found. The highest RRV was associated with places that have a proximity of 800 m to blight violations. With an RRV of 6.034, these places were six times more likely to experience a call for service for a mental health issue. As the RRVs may be directly compared, these areas were three times riskier for a mental health call for service when compared to places with an RRV of 2, such as proximity of 400 m to a larceny (RRV = 2.026). The risk factors with the highest values were blight violations (proximity, 800 m), assaults (proximity, 400 m) and larceny (proximity, 400 m), meaning that the places affected by these factors had the highest level of risk for mental health calls for service. The locations of demolitions, gun shops, homicides, and liquor outlets were unrelated to the occurrence of mental health calls for service. As can be seen in Table 2.1, the impact of the risk factors varied based on the specific type of mental health related call for service; that is, the RRVs for suicides and suicide attempts were different than those for non-violent mentally ill persons. For each type of mental health call for service, the 3 highest RRVs were bold in the table.

Table 2.1 Relative risk values, operationalization, and spatial influence for aggravating risk terrain model

	All mental health calls	Suicides and attempts	Violent, person with mental illness	Non-violent, person with mental illness
Assaults	**2.768 (P, 400)**	**3.146 (P, 400)**	**1.768 (D, 400)**	1.513 (D, 400)
Blight complaints	**6.034 (P, 800)**	1.353 (P, 400)	1.524 (P, 400)	1.642 (P, 400)
Burglaries	1.466 (P, 400)	1.331 (P, 400)	1.618 (P, 400)	1.353 (P, 400)
Car theft	1.658 (P, 400)	1.270 (D, 400)	1.695 (P, 400)	**1.832 (P, 400)**
Demolitions	X	X	X	X
Drug related	1.113 (D, 400)	X	X	1.235 (D, 400)
Family offenses	1.368 (P, 800)	**2.314 (P, 1200)**	1.185 (P, 400)	**2.336 (P, 1200)**
Gun shops	X	X	X	X
Homicides	X	X	1.135 (P, 800)	X
Larceny	**2.026 (P, 400)**	**2.225 (P, 400)**	**2.624 (P, 400)**	1.787 (D, 400)

(continued)

Table 2.1 (continued)

	All mental health calls	Suicides and attempts	Violent, person with mental illness	Non-violent, person with mental illness
Liquor licenses	X	1.394 (D, 1600)	X	X
Quality of life	1.517 (D, 400)	1.425 (D, 400)	**2.494 (P, 400)**	**3.105 (P, 400)**
Robbery	1.339 (D, 400)	1.412 (D, 400)	1.203 (D, 800)	1.501 (D, 400)
Sex assaults	1.272 (P, 400)	1.316 (P, 400)	1.199 (P, 400)	1.267 (P, 400)
Sex offenses	1.180 (P, 400)	1.193 (P, 400)	1.156 (P, 400)	X
Relative risk statistics				
Range of RRS	1–384.272	1–162.915	1–112.075	1–187.532
Mean	127.347	38.217	36.500	38.564
Stand. deviation	91.480	28.866	28.068	36.299
% >2 SD above mean	199 cells; 4.43% of study area	211 cells; 4.70% of study area	295 cells; 6.57% of study area	226 cells; 5.03% of study area

P = Proximity, D = Density

Relative Risk statistics are also presented in Table 2.1. Each of the 4490 cells of 400 × 400 m was assigned a relative risk score (RRS) ranging from 1 for the lowest risk cell to a maximum value. In the examination of all mental health related calls for service, the range of RRS was 1 to 384.272, which means that cells with an RRS of 384 have an expected rate of mental health calls for service that is 384 times *higher* than a place with a score of 1. The average RRV was 127.34 with a standard deviation of 91.48. There were 199 cells (or 4.43% of the study area) in which the RRS was greater than 2 standard deviation units above the mean, which implied that these cells had RRS of at least 310.30. Similar to the RRVs, the relative risk statistics varied based on the specific type of mental health related calls for service.

2.12 Protective Factors

Protective factors may be interpreted as a form of risk mitigation. That is, significant protective factors reduce the risk of future mental health related calls for service. Table 2.2 presents the summary results for the four protective factors tested in the model. As can be seen in Table 2.2, the protective influence of the potential factors was minimal at best. The proximity and/or density of parks was the only consistent protective factor for mental health related calls for service regardless of call type. As an example, the risk of a non-violent mentally ill call for service was

Table 2.2 Relative risk values, operationalization, and spatial influence for protective risk terrain model

	All mental health calls	Suicides and attempts	Violent, persons with mental illness	Non-violent, person with mental illness
Parks	2.048 (D, 1600)	1.620 (D, 3200)	1.991 (D, 1600)	1.851 (P, 400)
Places of worship	X	X	X	X
Recreation centers	X	1.140 (P, 2800)	X	X
Veterans centers	X	X	X	X
Relative risk statistics				
Range of RRS	1–2.048	1–1.846	1–1.991	1–1.851
Mean	1.927	1.653	1.876	1.788
Stand. deviation	0.336	0.259	0.317	0.223
% >2 SD above mean	0 cells; 0% of study area	0 cells; 0% of study area	0 cells; 0% of study area	0 cells; 0% of study area

reduced by nearly double in areas within 400 m of a park. None of the cells in the study area had a relative risk score that was greater than 2 standard deviations above the mean.

2.13 Discussion

The purpose of this study was to explore the geographic distribution of emergency calls for service for mental health related issues. As is the case with many social phenomena, the calls were not randomly distributed throughout the City of Detroit. Statistically significant hot and cold spots were identified for all mental health calls, suicides and suicide attempts, as well as people with mental illness who were violent and people with mental illness who were non-violent. The size and locations of the hot and cold spots varied based on the type of call. The total area for statistically significant hot spots (confidence >95%) for all mental health calls was 165.64 km^2. Conversely, the hot spot area for suicides and suicide attempts was 43.22 and 56.21 km^2 for hot spots involving people with mental illness who were violent. As the total area of the City is 660.25 km^2, the calls for service that pose the greatest risk to self (suicides) or others (people with mental illness who were violent) tended to concentrate in relatively small areas of the City. For suicides in particular, only 6.5% of the City's total area was identified as a hot spot. This finding can greatly assist in the development of targeted prevention efforts among social service agencies and community outreach centers to reduce the level of suicide in these areas.

As an example, based on the findings of the RTM analyses, places of worship were not found to be a protective factor for suicides. There were 49 worship centers located within the boundaries of the hot spots for suicides (see Fig. 2.5). If a 2 km buffer (1.43 miles) is added around the suicide hot spots, this number increases to 142, or approximately 61% of the worship centers in Detroit. This seems like a suicide prevention effort that could be relatively easy to incorporate. If residents knew that regardless of their faith a neighborhood worship center could provide them with emergency mental health services, there may be a direct impact on the number of suicides in the hot spot areas.

The results suggest that there were a number of factors that were related to the occurrence of calls for service for mental health issues, and the intensity of these factors varied based on the type of call for service. Some factors had little or no influence. First, there were two factors—the locations of demolitions and gun shops—that were not identified as risk factors for any of the types of mental health calls for service. One of the problems with the demolitions locations is that we do not know the status of the property once the removal process started. Is the home still standing and a magnet for vandalism, squatters, and crime, or is the property now a vacant lot being used for a community garden? The Detroit Land Bank Authority offers vacant side lots to neighboring homeowners for as little as $100

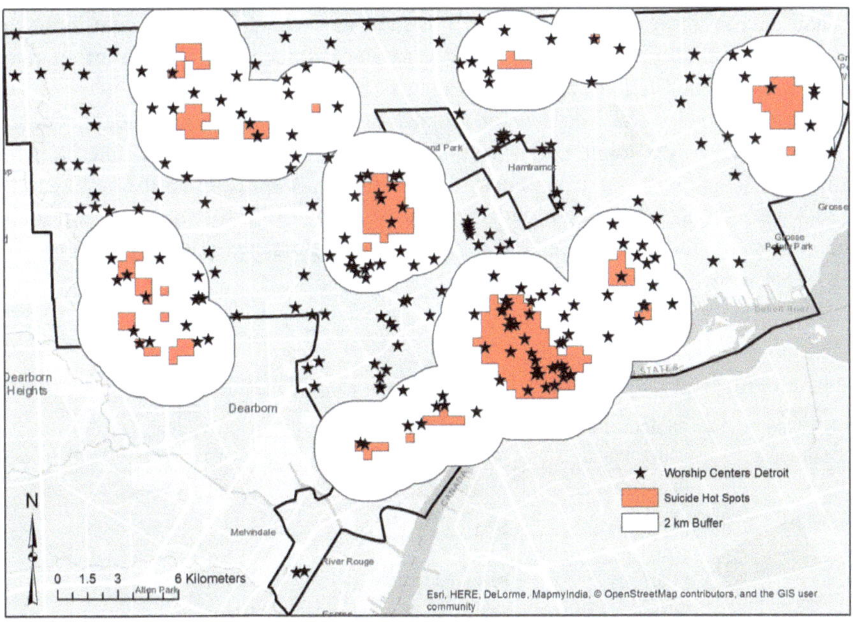

Fig. 2.5 Suicide hot spots and worship center locations

(www.buildingdetroit.org). It could be that a neighborhood is in much better condition after an abandoned home is on the demolition list and is in process for removal.

The locations of gun shops were not found to be related to mental health related calls for service, despite the link between firearms and suicide. The reader should be cautioned that this analysis included licensed gun dealers only; private points of sale are impossible to monitor. The State of Michigan does require that a potential buyer obtain a license from their local police department prior to the purchase of a handgun (Legislative Service Bureau, State of Michigan 2018). After purchase, the buyer must return for a firearm inspection from a private seller or dealer. It is difficult to estimate how many buyers go through the full legal process when purchasing a firearm from a private seller.

When examining the factors that did result in higher levels of risk, it is interesting to note that many of the more influential factors involved non-violent property crimes, blight violations, and quality of life offenses. Table 2.3 summarizes the top 5 risk factors for each type of mental health related call for service sorted by declining relative risk value. While the locations of simple and aggravated assaults were a consistent risk factor, so were larcenies, car thefts, and quality of life offenses. Larcenies involve the theft of property without force. Car thefts are also non-violent property crimes. Carjackings, which involve the use or threat of force, are classified as robberies and not car thefts. Family offenses, as defined in this research, may involve violence or non-violent acts of neglect. This finding is interesting given that the City of Detroit is consistently one of the most violent cities in the U.S. While crimes of violence do influence risk of calls for service for mental health issues, the relationship is not as strong as one might believe. Non-violent, quality of life issues have a greater influence on the risk of suicide, non-violent mental health, and violent mental health calls for service.

Protective factors had little to no impact on the risk for mental health related calls for service. Municipal parks were the only environmental feature that had any influence, which was minimal at best. The relative risk statistics in the aggravating model were much greater than what was found in the protective model. One of the challenges in identifying potential protective factors was finding where the resources were located.

Table 2.3 Top 5 relative risk factors for mental health classifications

All mental health calls	Suicides and attempts	Violent, person with mental illness	Non-violent, person with mental illness
Blight	Assaults	Larceny	Quality of life
Assaults	Family offenses	Quality of life	Family offenses
Larceny	Larceny	Assaults	Car theft
Car theft	Quality of life	Car theft	Blight
Quality of life	Robbery	Burglaries	Assaults

As is the case with risk factors, the selection of protective factors requires timely, accurate, and exhaustive location-based data. Consider the case of community gardens in Detroit. Given the number of vacant lots, urban gardens and farms have become a critical source of low-cost fruits and vegetables for Detroit residents. Working at the gardens has the potential to provide a number of activities related to mental health, i.e. social interaction, exercise, a sense of accomplishment, with community gardens related to certain positive outcomes (North Carolina State Extension, n.d.). Unfortunately, it is nearly impossible to identify the locations of these gardens. While estimates of the total number of gardens range from under 500 to nearly 1800 (Carmody 2018; Hill and Kuras 2017; Keep Growing Detroit 2018) only 30 community gardens were found on Google Earth and several inquiries for data to municipal and non-profit organizations were denied. While the potential risk reduction of community gardens on mental health would have been an interesting factor to include, it simply was not feasible. Similarly, accurate lists of mental health facilities, social service centers, food banks, free clinics and other community resources were difficult to identify. While Google Earth and other search engines were used, the consistency of the search results was poor. Interestingly, when the RTMDx software developers were contacted to verify the interpretation of the results, the authors were notified that no other study to date had been published using protective factors. Clearly, this is an important area of inquiry that merits further attention.

2.14 Limitations of the Study

The generalizability of the results beyond the City of Detroit must be mentioned. First, as stated previously, there are some characteristics of Detroit that make it a unique area of analysis including the population decline, abandoned and demolished buildings, and high rate of crime. Comparisons with cities with different demographics and growth trajectories may yield different results.

Second, this study relied heavily on official sources of data, such as calls for service and reported crimes. The Dark figure of crime, or crimes that go unreported to the police, is missing from the analysis. The crimes known to the police are viewed as only the tip of the iceberg, with vast amounts of criminal activity never officially counted (see Morgan and Truman 2018). People choose not to call the police to report a crime for a number of reasons. A citizen may fear reprisal by the offender if their identity as the complainant is somehow revealed; or a citizen might assume that someone else has already called the police. Others may feel that the police are not able to do anything about the crime or that the matter is not important enough to merit the attention of law enforcement. Regardless of the justification, many legitimate crimes go unreported and hence, do not show up in any official crime reports.

Third, the calls for service are based on the reports from citizens and/or police officers that an individual is in some sort of serious mental crisis that warrants emergency intervention from the police. This may or may not be the case. Additionally, no additional information on the disposition of the call is available. The individual of concern may have been released or transported to a hospital or other mental health assessment center. The gender, age, race, and ethnicity of the citizen were also unavailable for analysis.

Finally, the potential impact of the modifiable areal unit problem (MAUP) should be recognized. One of the problems when researching place is that the results are directly impacted by the areal unit selected for analysis—a different unit of analysis may yield different results (see, for example, Cutchin and Churchill 1999; Park and Peterson 2014). In the present study, the optimized hot spot analysis was based on the point locations of the calls for service. Alternatively, the calls for service could have been aggregated to a census block, block group, or tract, which would have allowed for the identification of hot spots using rates instead of points. Similarly, in the selection of place size and standard values in the RTMDx analyses, different place sizes could have impacted the results. It is important to keep the MAUP in mind and perhaps future researchers could attempt to replicate these findings using different units or analyses, such as spatial regression models.

Appendix: Data Descriptions

Layer	Source	Date accessed	Data link	Description
Blight violation notices	City of Detroit open data portal blight notifications	5/1/2019	https://data.detroitmi.gov/Property-Parcels/Blight-Violations/ti6p-wcg4	Blight violations notices from 9/7/2017–5/1/2019
Demolitions	City of Detroit open data portal Detroit demolitions	5/5/2019	https://data.detroitmi.gov/Property-Parcels/Detroit-Demolitions/rv44-e9di	Demolition Dates from 1/1/2014–5/5/2019
Gun dealers	Google Earth	5/5/2019		Includes all firearms dealers within city limits
Liquor licenses	City of Detroit open data liquor licenses	5/5/2019	https://data.detroitmi.gov/Public-Health/Liquor-Licenses/8hr2-enc6	Includes all active liquor licenses within city limits
Mental health calls	City of Detroit open data portal DPD: 911 calls for service	5/1/2019	https://data.detroitmi.gov/Public-Safety/DPD-911-Calls-for-Service-September-20-2016-Presen/wgv9-drfc	Includes suicides, suicide attempts, mental ill not violent, and mental violent

(continued)

(continued)

Layer	Source	Date accessed	Data link	Description
Parks	City of Detroit open data portal parks 2016	5/9/2019	https://data.detroitmi.gov/Fun/Parks-2016/yu9n-k8rd	Polygon shapefile downloaded from source
Places of worship	Google Earth	5/11/2019		Includes churches, synagogues, and mosques
Recreation centers	City of Detroit open data portal recreation centers	5/9/2019	https://data.detroitmi.gov/Fun/Recreation-Centers/8mnz-dib9	Point/address file downloaded from source
Reported crimes	City of Detroit open data portal DPD: all crime incidents	5/1/2019	https://data.detroitmi.gov/Public-Safety/DPD-All-Crime-Incidents-December-6-2016-Present/6gdg-y3kf	Includes all property, violent, and other criminal offenses
Veteran service centers	Google Earth/RTMx search	5/19/2019		Includes VA Medical Centers; VA Service Centers; and veterans support organizations

References

Abrutyn, S., & Mueller, A. S. (2014). The socioemotional foundations of suicide. *Sociological Theory, 32*(4), 327–351. https://doi.org/10.1177/0735275114558633.

Barnum, J., Caplan, J., Kennedy, L., & Piza, E. (2017). The crime kaleidoscope: A cross-jurisdictional analysis of place features and crime in three urban environments. *Applied Geography, 79,* 203–211. https://doi.org/10.1016/j.apgeog.2016.12.011.

Beyer, S. (2018, July 31). Why has detroit continued to decline? *Forbes.* https://www.forbes.com/sites/scottbeyer/2018/07/31/why-has-detroit-continued-to-decline/#232f13c43fbe. Accessed May 19, 2019.

Binelli, M. (2013). *Detroit city is the place to be* (1st ed.). New York, NY: Picador.

Bose, J., Hedden, S., Lipari, R. N., & Park-Lee, E. (2016). *Key substance use and mental health indicators in the United States: Results from the 2015 National Survey on Drug Use and Health.* Center for Behavioral Health Statistics and Quality. Substance Abuse and Mental Health Services Administration. Rockville, MD. https://www.samhsa.gov/data/sites/default/files/NSDUH-FFR1-2015/NSDUH-FFR1-2015/NSDUH-FFR1-2015.htm. Accessed on July 16, 2019.

Caplan, J., & Kennedy, L. W. (2010). *Risk terrain modeling manual: Theoretical framework and technical steps of spatial risk assessment.* Newark, NJ: Rutgers Center on Public Security.

Caplan, J., & Kennedy, L. (2013). *Risk terrain modeling diagnostics utility.* Newark, NJ: Rutgers Center on Public Security.

Caplan, J., & Kennedy, L. W. (2016). *Risk terrain modeling: Crime prediction and risk reduction.* Berkeley, CA: University of California Press.

Carmody, D. (2018, March 19). A growing city: Detroit's rich tradition of urban gardens plays an important role in the city's resurgence. *UrbanLand.* https://urbanland.uli.org/industry-sectors/public-spaces/growing-city-detroits-rich-tradition-urban-gardens-plays-important-role-citys-resurgence/. Accessed May 23, 2019.

Centers for Disease Control and Prevention. (2018a, January 26). *Learn about mental illness: Fast facts.* https://www.cdc.gov/mentalhealth/learn/index.htm also see https://www.cdc.gov/nchs/data/ahcd/namcs_summary/2014_namcs_web_tables.pdf. Accessed on July 16, 2019.

Centers for Disease Control and Prevention. (2018b, June 7). *Suicide rates rising across the U.S.* https://www.cdc.gov/media/releases/2018/p0607-suicide-prevention.html. Accessed June 14, 2019.

Chang, S., Sterne, J. A. C., Wheeler, B. W., Lu, T., Lin, J., & Gunnell, D. (2011). Geography of suicide in Taiwan: Spatial patterning and socioeconomic correlates. *Health and Place, 17*(2), 641–650. https://doi.org/10.1016/j.healthplace.2011.01.003.

City of Detroit. (n.d.). *Detroit's open data portal.* https://data.detroitmi.gov/. Accessed on July 16, 2019.

Cutchin, M., & Churchill, R. (1999). Scale, context, and causes of suicide in the United States. *Social Science Quarterly, 80*(1), 97–114.

Drawve, G., Thomas, S. A., & Walker, J. T. (2015). Bringing the physical environment back into neighborhood research: The unity of RTM for developing an aggregate neighborhood risk of crime measure. *Journal of Criminal Justice, 44,* 21–29. https://doi.org/10.1016/j.jcrimjus.2015.12.002.

Durkheim, E. (1857, 1951). *Suicide: A study in sociology.* Glencoe, IL: Free Press.

Esri. (2018). *How optimized hot spot analysis works.* https://pro.arcgis.com/en/pro-app/tool-reference/spatial-statistics/how-optimized-hot-spot-analysis-works.htm. Accessed May 27, 2019.

Faris, R. E., & Dunham, H. W. (1939). *Mental disorders in urban areas: an ecological study of schizophrenia and other psychoses.* Chicago, IL: The University of Chicago Press.

Federal Bureau of Investigation. (2018). *Crime in the United States 2017.* Washington D.C.: U.S. Department of Justice.

Hart, T. C., & Lersch, K. M. (2015). *Space, time, and crime* (4th ed.). Durham NC: Carolina Academic Press.

Hartz, S. M., Pato, C. N., Medeiros, H., et al. (2014). Comorbidity of severe psychotic disorders with measures of substance use. *JAMA Psychiatry, 71*(3), 248–254. https://doi.org/10.1001/jamapsychiatry.2013.3726.

Harvard School of Public Health. (2019). *Means matter: Firearm access is a risk factor for suicide.* https://www.hsph.harvard.edu/means-matter/means-matter/risk/. Accessed May 21, 2019.

Heffner, J. (2013). Statistics of the RTMDx utility. In J. Caplan & L. Kennedy (Eds.), *Risk terrain modeling diagnostics utility user manual (version 1.0).* Newark, NJ: Rutgers Center on Public Security.

Helbich, M. (2018a). Mental health and environmental exposures: An editorial. *International Journal of Environmental Research and Public Health, 15*(10), 2207. https://doi.org/10.3390/ijerph15102207.

Helbich, M. (2018b). Toward dynamic urban environmental exposure assessments in mental health research. *Environmental Research, 161,* 129–135. https://doi.org/10.1016/j.envres.2017.11.006.

Hempstead, K. (2006). The geography of self-injury: Spatial patterns in attempted and completed suicide. *Social Science and Medicine, 62*(12), 3186–3196. https://doi.org/10.1016/j.socscimed.2005.11.038.

Hill, A. B., & Kuras, A. (2017) *Detroit food metrics report 2017.* Detroit Food Policy Council and Detroit Health Department. https://www.dropbox.com/s/10yhmcym2lm68ap/DFMR17%20Report%20120717%20FINAL.pdf?dl=0. Accessed May 23, 2019.

Jane-Llopis, E., & Matytsina, I. (2006). Mental health and alcohol, drugs and tobacco: A review of the comorbidity between mental disorders and the use of alcohol, tobacco and illicit drugs. *Drug and Alcohol Review, 25,* 515–536. https://doi.org/10.1080/09595230600944461.

Jones, P. A. (2007). Researching the geography of mental wellbeing. *Journal of Mental Health, 16* (4), 439–443. https://doi.org/10.1080/09638230701482386.

Keep Growing Detroit. (2018). *Annual report.* http://detroitagriculture.net/wp-content/uploads/2018-KGD-Annual-Report_Final_Small.pdf. Accessed May 23, 2019.

Kirchner, T., & Shiffman, S. (2016). Spatio-temporal determinants of mental health and well-being: Advances in geographically-explicit ecological momentary assessment (GEMA). *Social Psychiatry and Psychiatric Epidemiology, 51*(9), 1211–1223. https://doi.org/10.1007/s00127-016-1277-5.

Lentz, J. (2009). *Spatial autocorrelation statistics.* http://jenniferalentz.info/Teaching/StudyGuides/SpatialAutocorrelation.pdf. Accessed May 27, 2019.

Livingston, J. (2016). Contact between police and people with mental disorders: A review of rates. *Psychiatric Services, 67*(8), 850–857. Retrieved from https://ps-psychiatryonline-org.ezproxy.lib.usf.edu/doi/pdf/10.1176/appi.ps.201500312.

Legislative Service Bureau, State of Michigan. (2018, April). *Firearms laws of Michigan.* https://www.legislature.mi.gov/Publications/Firearms.pdf. Accessed on July 15, 2019.

Mental Health Foundation. (2019). *Alcohol and mental health.* https://www.mentalhealth.org.uk/a-to-z/a/alcohol-and-mental-health Accessed May 21, 2019.

Morgan, R. E., & Truman, J. L. (2018). *Criminal victimization, 2017.* National Crime Victimization Survey, Bureau of Justice Statistics, https://www.bjs.gov/content/pub/pdf/cv17.pdf. Accessed on July 15, 2019.

National Institute of Mental Health. (2019, February). *Mental illn*ess. https://www.nimh.nih.gov/health/statistics/mental-illness.shtml. Accessed on July 15, 2019.

North Carolina State Extension. (n.d.). *Research regarding the benefits of community gardens.* https://nccommunitygardens.ces.ncsu.edu/nccommunitygardens-research/. Accessed on July 14, 2019.

Park, N., & Peterson, C. (2014). Suicide in happy places revisited: The geographical unit of analysis matters. *Applied Psychology: Health and Well-Being, 6*(3), 318–323. https://doi.org/10.1111/aphw.12030.

Philo, C. (2005). The geography of mental health: An established field? *Current Opinion in Psychiatry, 18*(5), 585–591. https://doi.org/10.1097/01.yco.0000179502.76676.c8.

Recker, N. L., & Moore, M. D. (2016). Durkheim, social capital, and suicide rates across US counties. *Health Sociology Review, 25*(1), 78–91. https://doi.org/10.1080/14461242.2015.1101703.

Rehkopf, D. H., & Buka, S. L. (2006). The association between suicide and the socio-economic characteristics of geographical areas: A systematic review. *Psychological Medicine, 36*(2), 145–157. https://doi.org/10.1017/S003329170500588X.

Shaw, C., & McKay, H. (1942). *Juvenile delinquency in urban areas.* Chicago, IL: University of Chicago Press.

Shueh, J. (2015, March 12). From debt to data: Detroit launches open data portal. *Government Technology.* https://www.govtech.com/data/From-Debt-to-Data-Detroit-Launches-Open-Data-Portal.html. Accessed May 20, 2019.

Stack, S. (2000a). Suicide: A 15-year review of the sociological literature. Part I: Cultural and economic factors. *Suicide & Life-Threatening Behavior, 30*(2), 145. Retrieved from https://www.ncbi.nlm.nih.gov/pubmed/10888055.

Stack, S. (2000b). Suicide: A 15-year review of the sociological literature. Part II: Modernization and social integration perspectives. *Suicide & Life-Threatening Behavior, 30*(2), 163. Retrieved from https://www.ncbi.nlm.nih.gov/pubmed/10888056.

Trgovac, A. B., Kedron, P. J., & Bagchi-Sen, S. (2015). Geographic variation in male suicide rates in the united states. *Applied Geography, 62,* 201–209. https://doi.org/10.1016/j.apgeog.2015.04.005.

Turner, H. A., Shattuck, A., Hamby, S., & Finkelhor, D. (2013). Community disorder, victimization exposure, and mental health in a national sample of youth. *Journal of Health and Social Behavior, 54*(2), 258–275. https://doi.org/10.1177/0022146513479384.

Vaughan, A. D., Hewitt, A. N., Hodgkinson, T., Andresen, M. A., & Verdun-Jones, S. (2018a). Temporal patterns of mental health act calls to the police. *Policing: A Journal of Policy and Practice, 13*(2), 172–185. https://doi.org/10.1093/police/pay060.

Vaughan, A. D., Hewitt, A. N., Andresen, M. A., Verdun-Jones, S. N., & Brantingham, P. (2019). The importance of gender in the spatial distribution of police interactions involving emotionally disturbed persons: An examination of call types. *Policing & Society: An International Journal of Research and Policy, 29*(2), 137–154. https://doi.org/10.1080/10439463.2017.1373110.

Vaughan, A. D., Ly, M., Andresen, M. A., Wuschke, K., Hodgkinson, T., & Campbell, A. (2018b). Concentrations and specialization of mental health-related calls for police service. *Victims & Offenders, 13*(8), 1153–1170. https://doi.org/10.1080/15564886.2018.1512539.

Weisheit, R. A., Facone, D. N., & Wells, L. E. (2006). *Crime and policing in rural and small-town America* (3rd ed.). Long Grove, IL: Waveland Press.

Wortley, R., & Mazerolle, L. (2008). *Environmental criminology and crime analysis.* Portland OR: Willan Publishing.

Wilson-Bates, F. (2008). *Lost in transition: How a lack of capacity in the mental health system is failing Vancouver's mentally ill and draining police resources.* Vancouver, BC, Canada: Vancouver Police Department.

Xie, Y., Gong, H., Lan, H., & Zeng, S. (2018). Examining shrinking city of Detroit in the context of socio-spatial inequalities. *Landscape and Urban Planning, 177,* 350–361. https://doi.org/10.1016/j.landurbplan.2018.03.002.

Yang, S. M., Gill, C., Kanewske, L. C., Thompson, P. S. (2018). Exploring police response to mental health calls in a nonurban area: A case study of Roanoke county, Virginia. *Victims & Offenders 13*(8), 1132–1152.

Chapter 3
Improving Estimates of the Quantity and Quality of Persons Involved in the Opioid Crisis

A. D. Vaughan

3.1 Introduction

The recent opioid epidemic has garnered a broad spectrum of attention from international-, national-, and state-policy makers, as well as academics, the media, patient groups and patient advocates.[1] It is worth highlighting that the present crisis did not emerge overnight. Much of the historical roots of opioid use and misuse is referenced by way of the medically supplied opioids narrative. In other words, the cause and subsequent solution to the opioid crisis is driven primarily by the health care system. Originally synthesized and industrially produced in Europe in the early 19th century, opioids were commonly used to treat acute pain from injuries and other recurrent minor pain (e.g., headaches) (Meldrum 2003). Morphine was used by military physicians to treat Civil War Veterans and, following the formal development of synthetic opioids in the late 1800s, opioids were used to treat acute pain (Rummans et al. 2018). Opioid use steadily increased in the early 1980s with many observers pointing to research that suggested that chronic pain could be safely managed with opioid medications that were not likely to lead to an addiction (Porter and Jick 1980). Such statements contradict what some practitioners had noted were addictive properties associated with opioids approximately 100 years earlier when morphine was first introduced to treat acute pain (Meldrum 2003).

Volumes of prescribed opioids exponentially increased in the mid-1990s through the combination of new synthetic opioids being produced and policy changes that

[1]Opioids represent a cluster of substances ranging from illicit drugs, such as heroin, to those that are prescribed in medical settings, which includes, but is not limited to: morphine, oxycodone (OxyContin), hydrocodone (Vicodin), oxymorphone, codeine, and fentanyl. Though not approved for human use, extremely powerful derivatives of opioids such as carfentanil have recently entered some drug markets.

A. D. Vaughan (✉)
Texas State University, San Marcos, USA
e-mail: a_v609@txstate.edu

K. M. Lersch and J. Chakraborty (eds.), *Geographies of Behavioural Health, Crime, and Disorder*, GeoJournal Library 126,
https://doi.org/10.1007/978-3-030-33467-3_3

reflected the notion that opioids were not likely to lead to severe addiction (Gilson and Joranson 2001). In the early 2000s, the opioid use narrative has followed the same upward trajectory with various spikes in increased usage through prescribing opioids to pain sufferers (Paulozzi et al. 2011). For example, a rich narrative about the history of pain clinics in certain jurisdictions highlights the immense quantities and other controlled substances that became available to the public, often "without medical evaluation or justification" (Dowell et al. 2016: 1877). More recently, additional varieties/analogs of opioids, such as those with abuse-deterrent properties, have been introduced to patients with some evidence to indicate the prescription opioid drug market has begun to show signs of shrinking (Pezalla et al. 2017). Conversely, there are countless reports from media, non-governmental organizations, practitioners and academics that indicate the rates of opioid-related deaths have risen exponentially across North America for the previous five to ten years (Rudd et al. 2016).

3.1.1 Scale of Impact

An unfortunate feature that parallels drug epidemics is that they often impact those with lower socioeconomic status (Brooks Dollar 2019). For example, the crack cocaine epidemic of the 1980s highlights the collateral effect of the lowered quality of life for those residing in poor minority communities in densely populated urban settings (Boggess and Bound 1997). In one study, the authors referred to this epidemic as "a social fire destroying the fabric of the inner city, its flame began to diminish by about 1989 as youths started to avoid its use" (Johnson et al. 1995: 290). Much of the social factors surrounding other drug epidemics are illustrated in the current opioid crisis. In some cases, opioid dependence has impacted the economy, housing markets, and the overall quality of life of opioid users and other members of the community (Aliprantis et al. 2019; Hagemeier 2018). Other studies highlight the drain on community services due to opioids including increased costs associated with victimization and law enforcement Wall et al. (2000) estimated that in 1996, the per capita cost from untreated opioid dependence ranged from $43 to $69; a per capita rate that is most certainly higher in the present day.

Given the nature of criminal law and lack of cohesive health policy for drug treatment, drug epidemics are also likely to intersect with the various layers of the criminal justice system. Violent crime is often correlated with drug use/trafficking. Although this is true in some instances, the correlation is often tied to the distribution and marketing of the drug because of the high rates of profit associated with trafficking in comparison to other street drugs available at the time (e.g., crack cocaine drug trafficking) (White and Gorman 2000). The use of the criminal justice system to enforce various drug policies, has, for the most part, been unable to make a meaningful impact on the drug trade. Some scholars suggest that drug epidemics proceed through various cycles of development (e.g., the characteristics of drug users and distributers change over the course of the epidemic) and "contrary to popular belief, they will not continue rampantly unless checked by exogenous factors, such as law enforcement" (Hamid 1992: 345). Regardless of this notion, "the war on drugs" and other conservative policy lenses to drug use in many Westernized nations has led to a copious amount of taxpayer funds being dedicated to law enforcement efforts, prosecution, and incarceration of drug users and low-level distributors. Decades of "zero-tolerance" drug policy have led to many settings having a larger than expected proportion of inmates having addictions and other substance use problems. For example, Carpentier et al. (2018) highlight that the proportion of the general population that has ever used cocaine varies between 0.3 and 6.8%, with approximately 2 and 43% of prisoners reporting cocaine use at any time outside prison.

In many jurisdictions, opioid users are subject to decades-old zero-tolerance drug policies. Local police services enforce these policies, which is then followed by criminal courts processing drug users (and traffickers). Lengthy, and at times mandatory, minimum prison sentences are commonplace, with the result being an overpopulation present in all levels of correctional facilities. In general, correctional facilities were never intended to provide any form of treatment to prisoners, and there is often no guarantee that treatment will be available (Chandler et al. 2009). Conversely, from a public health perspective, the history of opioid use and how it has evolved as a primary component to how "pain" is conceptualized and subsequently managed, results in a different type of drug crisis that does not mirror the patterns illustrated in the crack cocaine and methamphetamine crises of late 20th century (Brooks Dollar 2019). For example, modern conceptualizations of medical practitioners and how society, more broadly, responds to pain goes beyond just treating acute physical injuries, and now encompasses chronic pain which may be used as a refuge for psychological trauma (Dasgupta et al. 2018). Thus, many have argued that the current epidemic's foundation, was born out of decades of medical/pharmaceutical practice, fortified through more restrictive prescription practices, and amplified through increased availability of illicit opioids.

3.1.2 Data Considerations

Thus far, the reader has been presented with a rather stark narrative of where opioid use began, and the current state of affairs in not only the United States, but other Westernized nations as well, such as: Canada (Fischer et al. 2018), the United Kingdom (Giraudon et al. 2013), and Australia (Leong et al. 2009). The pervasiveness of the opioid crisis across different facets of life presents scholars, policy makers and practitioners with the opportunity to understand the crisis at different stages. In all stages, there are a variety of potentially valuable data points. Some data points are used extensively (and for good reason) whereas other data points are less well-known. On the more "cited" end of the spectrum of data that speaks to the opioid crisis is mortality statistics.

Arguably, mortality statistics are the most useful source of information that should guide jurisdictions on how they should best respond to the problem to have a relatively immediate impact on saving lives. From a public health perspective, basic mortality data on the means and cause of death are vital to assess patterns and risks associated with death due to opioid-use. Among a host of other things, counts of opioid-caused overdose (OD) deaths will be imperative for testing if an intervention plan is effective at saving lives (Irvine et al. 2019; Rando et al. 2015). Not surprisingly, the seriousness surrounding opioid-related deaths in certain North American jurisdictions has resulted in calls-for-action from interest groups such as the distribution of more products that are engineered to reverse opioid-related ODs (Babcock et al. 2017).

In addition to front-line or street-level data sources, more "upstream" data sources exist. Understanding the nature of opioid use prior to an OD will inevitably capture a larger portion of the opioid-using population. Hospitals routinely collect such data. For example, a patient may present to the emergency department (ED) on their own volition for withdrawal symptoms associated with opioid use. In other cases, overdose patients will present to the ED via an ambulance and some of these patients will be revived by medical staff. As previously mentioned, the healthcare system also captures information on changes in patterning of opioid prescription. The 2016 United States Centre for Disease Control and Prevention (CDC) policy guideline for prescribing opioids in primary care settings is a significant step in the direction of reducing over-prescription of opioids. Of course, one cannot assume that all physicians over prescribed opioids to begin with, nor can the assumption be made that all physicians will adhere to these guidelines.

And of course, there is the group of opioid users who are not well-captured in traditional databases. These patients have a history of opioid use but are not classified as being addicted nor physically dependent on the drug. In other words, because their drug use is sporadic and not tied to any sort of treatment plan, an official record of their opioid use is likely to be absent. Knowledge of this "hidden" cohort is vital to ensuring practitioners understand the factors that are likely to lead to a shift to more problematic opioid use in the future. To generate this knowledge various methodological approaches such as self-report data may be used to measure the extent of the opioid crisis.

3.1.3 Aim of the Chapter

The collection of diverse sets of data is advantageous because it produces a multifaceted foundation of a given phenomenon, and thus provides a more balanced evidence-base from which to generate policy, programing, and other initiatives. When combined with innovative methodologies, such as those used to approximate and predict the population size, the ability to more accurately respond to the current and future levels of the opioid crisis is possible. The current rate of opioid use in many Westernized nations demands these broad lenses to ensure policy frameworks are holistic in nature by addressing the needs and spectrum of risks associated with opioid use (Morrow et al. 2019). Unfortunately, stakeholders rarely have access to "data on drug use, treatment, and public safety outcomes [as these] are managed in different agencies and are often not integrated in a comprehensive way that facilitates the needs of public safety and public health" (Christie et al. 2017: 58).

The current chapter provides a multifaceted framework of data and research methodologies for the purposes of improving prevalence estimates of all opioid users. Improvements in the calculation of the size and nature of opioid users in a given community is vital for the development of programs, policies, and formal evaluations of these efforts. Four broad areas of data and methodological approaches are vital to make these improvements: (A) OD death data; (B) Community data; (C) prescription data; and (D) predictive/modelling techniques. These data streams are presented in order of urgency with OD data and other emergency data highlighting imminent health concerns. Conversely, other non-emergency data and predictive modelling are more "upstream" data sources whereby in theory, these data exist prior to an emergency.

3.2 Data and Methodological Approaches

(A) *OD Death Data*

Hedegaard et al. (2018: 4) indicate that the rate of overdose deaths due to synthetic opioids (e.g., fentanyl) in the United States has "increased on average by 8% per year from 1999 through 2013 and by 71% per year from 2013 through 2017." In addition, one cannot overlook the recent exponential increase in the death rate from 2016 to 2017 (i.e., 45.2%) resulting in a tally of 47,600 opioid-OD deaths in 2017 (Scholl et al. 2019). Though not with the same exponential-level of increase, other OD deaths have also been steadily increasing for the past 15 years with other natural (e.g., morphine) and semi-synthetic opioids (e.g., oxycodone).

As is common in other health epidemics, risk of OD death is not uniformly distributed over space, time, and by population. For example, in the United States, middle-aged persons (i.e., 25–54) are at the highest risk of OD deaths with a lower risk being observed for youth and the elderly (Hedegaard et al. 2018). Geographically speaking, aggregate rates of OD deaths are generally comparable. For example, in 2014, the Northeast, Midwest, South, and Western regions of the United States had OD death rates per 100,000 population ranging from 13.7–16.1 (Rudd et al. 2016). As the areal unit of analysis under investigation becomes more disaggregated, more telling clusters of OD deaths begin to emerge. Known as the epicenters for the opioid crisis in their respective countries, Vancouver, British Columbia (Scheuermeyer et al. 2019) and Cabell County, West Virginia (Merino et al. 2019) have had exceedingly high OD death rates. For example, Vancouver had 215 fatal ODs in 2016, a rate three times higher than the historical average. In 2015, the OD death rate in Cabell County was 140 per 100,000 persons, a rate approximately 10 times higher than the national average (approximately 13.5/100,000) (Babcock et al. 2017). Though speaking to a subset of addicted opioid users, Marshall et al. (2018: 85) point out what is seemingly obvious in that "opioid addiction is a disease that does not recognize geographic boundaries, and treating this epidemic will require expanding intervention areas and including a more diverse population than once prior thought."

At the neighborhood and street-segment level, research indicates further spatial concentration. For example, Marshall et al. (2018) explored the relationship between socioeconomic status and residential demographics with opioid OD death concentrations via ZIP code in Orange County, California. Although the researchers found that "ZIP codes with higher opioid-related death concentration appear to be prevalent among many affluent communities along the Pacific coast… [the] geographic distribution does not appear to have a particular epicenter within one particular ZIP code, but rather more of a diffuse distribution" (2018: 83). At the street-segment level, Carter et al. (2019) found that opioid-related OD deaths in Indianapolis were highly concentrated. For example, using 500 m^2 block segments, the authors found that 5% of block segments contained "53.5% of any opioid death, 57.5% of any illicit opioid death, 64.8% of any prescription opioid death, and 49.0% of paramedic drug overdose calls" (Carter et al. 2019: 174). In response to this known geographic concentration, various programs have been introduced to prevent OD deaths. Through an investigation of the patient-specific and contextual characteristics (Amram et al. 2019), researchers found an inverse relationship between lower density opioid agnostic treatment (OAT) facilities (i.e., methadone clinics) within a neighborhood, and an increased rate of OD.[2] In other words, the location of treatment programs is important to not only delivering services but also saving potential lives.

<u>OD data caveat</u>

At the outset, data on death associated with opioid uses should be easily captured over space, time, and by patient. Indeed, evaluations of surrounding naloxone distribution and other urgent lifesaving policies are likely to have some understanding of the baseline OD opioid death rate in a given jurisdiction to determine if said policy saves lives (Irvine et al. 2019; Rees et al. 2019). Though these initiatives intended to provide support for the general population and emergency responders are important for saving lives, one of the major challenges is the quality of the death data. In general, the methodology for generating death data is place-specific and may be inconsistent. Caution should be used when interpreting opioid-related death rates (Lisa and Jessica 2018). For instance, in some locations, medicolegal death investigations (MDI) and certifications of overdose deaths are completed by a medical examiner or forensic examiners. This is a medically trained group, and as such, it should be expected that their expertise will limit the amount

[2]OAT provide patients with long-acting opioids (e.g., methadone and suboxone) to prevent withdrawal symptoms from other opioids that a patient may be using (e.g., heroin).

of variability in MDI. In other locations, coroners perform MDI. Often coroners are not required to have medical training, and, in the United States, coroners are elected positions. In contrast, medical examiners are appointed by the governing authority of a given jurisdiction. Scholars have argued for increased consistency and accuracy of OD death investigations with some suggesting that all MDI "should be performed or supervised by a board certified forensic pathologist" (National Research Council 2009: 268).

A lack of standardized MDI procedures inevitably leads to errors in MDI data. Coupled with some deaths involving multiple drugs that may have been associated with an OD (Ogbu et al. 2015), for a variety of reasons, it should be expected that a certain proportion of MDI will be misclassified. There will also be a certain degree of attrition from all cases that are reported to the coroner/medical examiner's office and those that are accepted. In many cases, a formal death investigation will not take place. In these cases, a certain proportion of opioid-related OD deaths will be undocumented, resulting in no death certificate, or a death certificate will be produced but the cause of death will be "undetermined" (Kelsall and Bowes 2016). For opioid deaths, the estimate of how many undocumented cases is unknown, but a recent study suggests that this missing data is substantial:

> States may be markedly underestimating the effect of opioid related overdose deaths because of incomplete cause-of-death reporting. Potentially 70,000 opioid-related, unintentional overdose deaths from 1999 through 2015 have been missed because of incomplete reporting, indicating that the opioid overdose epidemic may be worse than it appears. (Buchanich et al. 2018: 430)

Discourse around illicit and prescription opioids and their relationship to OD deaths is often independent and resulting policies may reflect this narrative. There is a lack of consensus to whether MDI investigations can distinguish between the underlying type of opioid that caused death. On the one hand, some studies indicate the ability to differentiate deaths caused by prescription opioids only, those involving illicit opioids only, and both prescription and illicit opioids (Mattson et al. 2018). On the other hand, some scholars indicate that "illicitly manufactured fentanyl cannot be distinguished from prescription fentanyl in death certificate data" (Rudd et al. 2016: 1323).

The status of OD death data is further complicated when including the misclassified/unclassified cases. In the United States, for example, scholars have found troubling patient-level demographic trends (gender, race, age, education), as well as geographic and economic trends. Boslett et al. (2019) found high levels of unclassified cases in Alabama, Arkansas, Indiana, Louisiana, Mississippi, Missouri, and Pennsylvania and speculated that these high case counts may be related to high rates of coroner MDI in these states. Economically speaking, the authors found that in addition to that the exiting OD death may be underestimated in women, "poorer counties may be marked by higher rates of underreported opioid overdoses, masking an even deeper crisis in poverty-stricken areas than we currently realize" (Boslett et al. 2019: 8).

The variety of MDI investigation practices in Western nations along with the complex relationship some users have between prescription and illicit opioids further emphasize the need for some degree of standardization in MDI practice. This consistency in practice is vital to reduce misclassified cases as well as to ensure that all segments of the opioid-using population receive a high-quality MDI if their usage results in an OD death. Holding all the shortcomings of the MDI data in check, of the OD death data that do exist, the narrative is troubling. For many communities, the epidemic has not subsided and has only worsened with no foreseeable end to the crisis.

(B) *Community Data*

Although it may appear obvious, not all ODs result in death. According to Melton and Melton (2019: 165), the rate of nonfatal overdose cannot be precisely measured… there are 20–30 nonfatal overdoses to every fatal overdose. While 115 people dying daily in the US from drug overdose is shocking enough, the almost 2 million nonfatal overdoses in 2017 are destroying lives, weakening communities, and overburdening the healthcare system. Emergency responders (Rando et al. 2015) and peer groups (Bennett et al. 2018) may also play a significant role in saving the lives of opioid users that have OD. As one shifts the focus away from MDI data and towards those related events that did not result in a fatality, the potential "net" of data sources begins to widen. This antecedent data to opioid-related deaths are important as they provide researchers, policy makers and practitioners a highly relevant narrative about a theoretically larger, and perhaps qualitatively unique, high-risk segment of opioid users.

The focus of this section will continue to address high-risk opioid users but through potential data sources that are found within official records management data that are generated by community service providers. Of interest will be data sources that reference the illicit drug market and those involved in emergency health services.

Illicit drug market data

In the decades that it has taken for the opioid crisis to develop, much has been learned about the current state of the illicit opioid drug market. In some jurisdictions, the illicit opioid market is highly toxic. Various methodologies have been used to explore the toxicity in the evolving opioid market including testing from border seizures, confiscated drugs, postmortem toxicology and front-line drug testing (Tyndall 2018). Of interest is the ability for service providers to use novel techniques to detect clandestine-lab-generated opioids in the illicit drug market. From a healthcare perspective, mass spectrometer has shown to be able to be reliable at identifying the precise type of opioid analogue in a given sample (Armenian et al. 2018). Unfortunately, mass spectrometer testing is often only available in laboratories, and local hospitals may not be able to provide efficient real-time testing. Recent advancements in portable/mobile mass spectrometer allow for testing and detection in these settings (Lawton et al. 2017), though the ability to expand these programs is extremely costly. A more affordable option to detect the toxicity of opioids in the illicit market is with self-administered testing strips. In some areas, test strips are becoming increasingly available via online purchasing, despite the lack of peer-reviewed evidence to suggest that the strips accurately identify fentanyl (McGowan et al. 2018).

The role of the criminal justice system in the illicit drug market is often to combat the supply and trafficking of these substances. With almost half a century of enforcement, the impact of criminal law and policing efforts on the illicit drug market has been minimal. Some scholars have suggested that although drug markets may be pressured by enforcement to change, in general, these ever-changing markets "cannot be effectively controlled through enforcement of the criminal law" (May and Hough 2004: 560). In tandem with various policing efforts, scholars have been able to highlight various patterns in the drug market. For example, in a study of the spatial concentration of drug activity in Seattle, scholars found that there was a high degree of concentration at the street-segment level (Hibdon et al. 2017). As expected, these spatial patterns varied over time. Police enforcement priorities, along with the intricate relationship between drugs and crime, may result in more (or less) police response to a given area and dilute the amount of concentration of a given drug market in that area. Some research has suggested that "crackdowns" on drug use displace the problem to adjacent jurisdictions which may impact new users in areas that lack the necessary programing to respond to and prevent drug use (Wood et al. 2004). As Curtis and Wendel (2000: 144) explain, "the developmental trajectories of drug distribution and consumption vary considerably from neighborhood to neighborhood. Neighborhoods are complex, multidimensional entities where structural constraints and micro factors intersect to form culturally diverse social fabrics."

Front-line law enforcement efforts are arguably the best link to estimating the quantity of illicit opioids in the market. At the local level, law-enforcement conducts clandestine lab seizures, which may contain drugs other than illicit opioids (Peck et al. 2019), place attention on tracking pill pressing machines (Bronskill 2018; Christie et al. 2017), and could be involved in naloxone distribution (where available) (Rando et al. 2015). Law enforcement efforts at border crossings are also useful proxy for the volume of police-detected opioids in the market. Gladden (2016) found there to be a correlation between seized shipments of fentanyl and synthetic opioid overdoses. Large port cities are often a destination for illicit opioids, so it is unsurprising that a large quantity of fentanyl and other opioids remain in these locations for distribution to the local opioid users. In other cases, the culprit for high degrees of fentanyl concentration in areas away from major ports-of-entry such as the Northeast and Midwest regions of the United States are less well-known. Ciccarone (2019: 3) highlights that "a demand or culturally driven event, such as through entrepreneurial or individual internet purchases, would more likely have led to a more even geographic spread" of illicit fentanyl. Traditional policing efforts in the online market are often even more limited. Dark web markets are often a crucial source of fentanyl and other synthetic opioids, and in some cases, Tor web browsing allows for nearly anonymous payment and shipping (Popper 2019).

Existing police RMS data provide an additional opportunity to understand the opioid crisis. In addition to analyzing geospatial patterns (Carter et al. 2019), other scholars have considered the diversion of prescribed opioids into the illicit market. For instance, Rodwell et al. (2010: 10) found "some evidence that prescription medicines are being diverted from the medical system through prescription forgeries and theft-related offences." An additional feature often contained within police RMS systems is the name of parties involved in an event. Not all police events result in a formal RMS file, but if a file has been completed, the names of the victim and offender, for example, should be noted, and in reference to a local master name index (Plecas et al. 2011). The ability for the police to identify offenders of opioid manufacturing and trafficking is paramount in responding to the crisis through the enforcement of law. In addition, the identification of frequent users of opioids that are also contained within police RMS systems is of great value for public health. As Kilmer et al. (2015: 232) suggest, "the number of frequent or heavy users is a better measure of the threat to population health than simple prevalence, since most of the health problems are associated with those who are dependent or who abuse these drugs." Rarely are police RMS data or other police databases analyzed to identify patterns in opioid use not only for those who are addicted but for all types of users. As such, there is great potential to computationally reconstruct the patterns in the illicit drug market with existing police data.

Given their enforcement role of drug laws, police services are often well-positioned to provide data on those quantities of opioids as well as those involved in the trafficking and consumption of said drugs. At the same time, the police have a duty to keep persons safe in the community, which includes opioid users. Given their relationship with a subgroup of the opioid using population, the police are well-positioned to help identify high-risk opioid users that may benefit from a referral for acute treatment and short-term detoxification services (Schiff et al. 2017).

Emergency responder and hospital data

A vast quantity of resources is funneled into the emergency healthcare system through EDs and pre-hospital settings. Naloxone distribution is arguably the most widely discussed in the media and depending on the jurisdiction, a variety of emergency responders and laypersons may be equipped with the overdose reversing drug (Davis et al. 2014; Lambdin et al. 2018).

Notwithstanding the myriad factors that can lead to an overdose (Schneider et al. 2019) and impact the development of a local illicit drug market, there is evidence to suggest that rural communities are particularly vulnerable given their "remoteness" to treatment services. As a result, naloxone distribution in these less densely populated areas may be more common. For example, in a study of Wyoming paramedics, Kilwein et al. (2019: 3) state: "EMS providers in remote areas with longer transport times and less law enforcement backup reported titrating naloxone more often."

Monitoring the number of naloxone doses provided to emergency responders and laypersons in a given jurisdiction offers stakeholders with an additional data source. Of great interest would be to compare naloxone usage with MDI data to determine the relative effectiveness of naloxone. Given the rising cost of naloxone (Gupta et al. 2016), determining how much naloxone should exist in a community to counteract the risk of OD is also vital to effectively and efficiently combating the opioid crisis.[3] In theory, a government authority could track naloxone purchases and use-rate in emergency responders, but as jurisdictions expand the access to pharmacies and laypersons, the ability to measure the amount of naloxone in the market will be more difficult. For example, in a recent study in Texas, researchers found that although pharmacies generally follow the state-enforced policy for increased naloxone availability in the state, only 76.4% of sampled pharmacies had naloxone available and 83.7% would dispense the drug without a prescription (Evoy et al. 2018).

Hospitals and EDs have been particularly hard hit by the opioid crisis. For example, many ODs are eventually diverted to the ED for a more thorough medical evaluation and potential treatment. As such, it is no surprise that rates of opioid-related presentations have paralleled the trajectory of the opioid crisis over the past ten years (Guy et al. 2018; Lovegrove et al. 2019; Moe et al. 2018). A recent CDC publication highlights the immense scale that the opioid crisis has on front-line EDs. In addition to high concentrations of ED presentations in the Southwest, Midwest, and Western regions of the United States, “a total of 142,557 ED visits occurred between July 2016 through September 2017, and the prevalence of suspected opioid overdose ED visits substantially increased between 29.7 and 34.5% from third quarter 2016 to third quarter 2017” (Vivolo-Kantor et al. 2018: 282). This tremendous growth in ED visits is likely to extend to even higher estimates when accounting for other factors. For example, co-occurring substances, such as benzodiazepines, may amplify the effects of an opioid-related respiratory failure (Jones and McAninch 2015). This complexity is amplified even further when considering the underlying “source” of a patient’s opioid presentation to the ED. Research suggests that in the United States, prescription opioids were found to be involved in 67.8% of all overdose presentations to the ED (Yokell et al. 2014). The data for their study precedes the current opioid epidemic by several years, but illicit (e.g., heroin), unspecified opioids, and multiple opioids were associated with a relatively high number of ED presentations: 16.1%, 13.4%, and 2.7%, respectively.

Patients often present to the ED when in a state of crisis which may lead to poor connectivity to treatment plans. However, some studies highlight that EDs often play a crucial gatekeeping role in preventing repeated overdoses and referring patients to treatment services (Duber et al. 2018; Skinner et al. 2009). For example,

[3]Gupta et al. (2016: 2214) state that in 2016 in the United States, naloxone delivered in nasal format costs $150. The same two-dose auto-injector version of naloxone “was priced at $690 in 2014 but is $4500 today, a price increase of more than 500% in just over 2 years”.

ED referrals to opioid agonist treatment such as methadone have been shown to be somewhat successful in effectively treating patients who are dependent on opioids (D'Onofrio et al. 2015).

Access to health insurance in jurisdictions without publicly funded health insurance programs often becomes a significant factor in who does and does not present to the ED. Choi et al. (2019: 16) found that persons with low socioeconomic status (i.e., Medicaid beneficiaries) "were more likely to utilize the ED and be repeat ED utilizers compared to commercially insured patients." The complexity of the nexus between treatment and presenting to the ED is further amplified when considering health insurance. Along with important sex differences, financial barriers to accessing opioid agonist programs may result in an influx of a segment of the opioid-using population presenting to the ED (John and Wu 2019). Synchronized data systems that share pertinent ED data is crucial to early intervention for high risk patients, particularly when first time exposure to opioids through the ED for acute pain, for example, has been found to be correlated with future problematic opioid use (Butler et al. 2016). The results from Axeen et al. (2018: 665) indicates another potentially high risk group of patients:

> EDs might dispense disproportionate amounts of prescriptions to high-risk users. The notion is that opioid-addicted individuals move from ED to ED, taking advantage of the lack of provider continuity to acquire large quantities of opioids. However, we found that high-risk opioid users received only a fraction of their opioids from EDs.

It is unclear as to whether this subgroup of opioid users is aware of the data sharing loopholes that exists between EDs/health authorities. Building data sharing agreements between different EDs that are housed in different insurance networks and/or health authorities (if only to identify opioid users who "shop" different EDs for opioids) would allow for the identification of a subgroup of high-risk nomadic opioid users.

(C) *Prescription Data*

Of the myriad legal, social, economic, and health-based factors that have led to the current opioid crisis, prescriptions of opioids dominate the discourse. Determining how much of the crisis is caused by prescribing practices will often yield a high degree of variability in the data. Like other data sources in healthcare and criminal justice, obtaining access to recent data on prescriptions is vital in order to effectively surveil the opioid crisis. Unfortunately, because prescription data is tied to privacy protection and in some jurisdictions, linked to powerful corporations, no data may be made available to policy makers. If data has been made available, there may be a significant lag in gaining access to it. A recent court decision in the United States highlights the value of prescription patterning data while also highlighting the time lag issue. The recent Federal Government database that monitors other pertinent information, the volume and location of prescription opioids, as well as the prescribing physician and where the prescription was filled, was released in 2019. According to the Washington Post investigative reporters, some 76 billion prescription pain pills were manufactured and shipped to pharmacies across the United States from 2006 to 2012 (Hingham et al. 2019). Timely access to prescription data is fundamental to providing public health officials with the necessary evidence base to surveil the opioid crisis (or any drug crisis for that matter).

Intertwined in the prescription narrative are changes to policy and practice which cannot be understated. As mentioned previously, in 2016, the CDC updated its guidelines for prescribing opioids for chronic pain suggesting a variety of changes in medical practice such as determining when to initiate or continue opioids for chronic pain, the type of opioid (e.g., immediate-release vs. long-acting opioids), the dosage and duration of treatment, and evaluation strategies for adjusting the treatment plan (Dowell et al. 2016). Unfortunately, some scholars have suggested that as prescription volumes decreased, an expected feedback loop emerged. For example, between 2005 and 2010, increases were observed in illicit opioid users shifting to drugs like heroin instead (Cicero et al. 2017). Other considerations that have been raised by clinicians regarding the new guideline includes, but is not limited to, "the time required to discuss alternative forms of pain control, the difficulty in obtaining reimbursement for alternatives, how to address opioid tapering, and concerns with the prescribing guideline for specific forms of pain" (Christie et al. 2017: 48).

Much of the potential significance of patterns within ED data, pharmaceutical data and physician practices such as the treatment plans for patients with chronic/acute pain are often buried behind privacy legislation, confidentiality agreements and other essential policies that are designed to safeguard sensitive health information. A potential solution for future work to understand the spectrum of opioid users should be to develop mechanisms to allow for the sharing of sensitive information through data stewards or an approved third-party representative that can ensure that the data management and dissemination adheres to privacy law. As an example, The Province of British Columbia in Canada has gradually made such a system of data sharing available to public health officials and academics to develop more comprehensive narratives on a given health phenomenon. Data stewards from different service providers work with Population Data BC (PopData) as a third party entity to facilitate interdisciplinary research on the determinants of human health, well-being and development (Population DataBC 2019).

In relation to the current opioid crisis, a recent study highlights the ability for data sharing platforms to enable a more complete understanding of the opioid epidemic such as being able to identify high-risk subgroups, and patterning of healthcare system usage. Coupled with the Provincial Medical Health Officer's announcement that the opioid crisis was a public health emergency, MacDougall et al. (2019) were able to integrate a myriad pertinent data sources into their model, including data from the provincial ambulance service, drug and poison calls from the public, coroners reports, ED presentations, discharge records, billing records to BC's universal health insurance program, and records of all prescriptions of pharmaceuticals made in the province.

(D) *Predictive/Modelling Techniques*

Though the evidence from prescription opioids is compelling as to a primary root cause to the present-day crisis, the mixture of illicit and legal opioids is not always salient. In fact, it is not entirely clear as to whether illicit opioid drug markets were created because users demanded them or if it was imposed on them. Mars et al. (2019) highlight the need to understand what drives any changes in the illicit drug market and that without this knowledge, policy interventions will be limited in their degree of effectiveness. The authors go on to state that "any determination of whether the current wave of fentanyl in the opioid street supply is demand- or supply-led relies on understanding sales methods, its reception among users and market conditions in specific national contexts" (Mars et al. 2019: 778).

The need to gather a larger spectrum of data is evident for those who are involved in the illicit manufacturing of opioids to determine what factors create and perpetuate this type of market. In addition, the flourishing prescription market for opioids is not entirely independent of the illicit market creating a complex network of opioids, distributors, and a spectrum of users ranging from those who use the drug recreationally to those with an opioid addiction and everyone in between. Innovative techniques that have emerged in recent years provide stakeholders with an ability to estimate the quantity of opioids in the market. For instance, scholars have scientifically tested untreated wastewater for the presence or absence of drugs (van Nuijs et al. 2011). Referred to as sewage epidemiology, this multi-disciplinary approach can generate a drug profile specific to opioids in hotspots in a given jurisdiction. In a recent study conducted in Northeast Spain, researchers estimated heroin consumption of 138 mg/day per 1000 residents with 61 mg/day per 1000 inhabitants aged between 15 and 64 years (Postigo et al. 2010). One advantage of wastewater studies to estimate the volume of opioids in the market is the ability to triangulate the results with other data sources such as prescription sales, syringe distribution data and self-report data (Been et al. 2015).

Self-report data is common in studies about drug use. One major advantage of this methodological approach over traditional methods such as MDI or prescription data is the ability to identify persons who have not been formally captured by traditional data collection mechanisms. The fact that a certain proportion of opioid users will not have a healthcare record related to opioids (e.g., prescriptions, hospital visits), or have had any contact with other service providers who also capture information on the opioid market (e.g., police RMS systems) results in a gap in knowledge. The opioid crisis has a broad impact over the population so national surveys on opioid use (Han et al. 2017), as well as those in subgroups of the population such as those serving in the military (Toblin et al. 2014), is very important. In fact, through self-report data, Winkelman et al. (2018) identified that opioid users often have other health problems and they are likely to have criminal justice system involvement. Self-report data is particularly useful for capturing emerging subsets of opioid users such as adolescents. For example, to study the opioid epidemic using patterns in the youth population, McCabe and colleagues collected self-report drug use data over a 17-month period from all middle and high school students in 2 public school districts in the Detroit metropolitan area.

When the criterion for inclusion in the sample involves stigmatized and/or illegal behavior, some individuals may be understandably reluctant to be interviewed or provide any form of self-report data. Samples of opioid users that intersect with multiple systems (Winkelman et al. 2018) often means making some form of sampling decisions to mirror that what is in the population, while accounting for some degree of sampling error. One method that goes beyond traditional sampling techniques to produce estimates of the size and nature of a population is capture-recapture techniques. Though the underlying mathematics varies, the methodology generally involves a minimum of two series of data collection: (1) capturing and marking the first sample, and (2) recapturing at a later point in time to make notation of the difference between the captures (Frischer et al. 1991). Capture-recapture techniques have been used in a variety of settings, including estimating the size of illicit drug markets (Bouchard 2007). Recently, it has been implemented to estimate and describe the number of persons who inject drugs in Cabell County, West Virginia (Allen et al. 2019). The technique has also been used to estimate that the proportion of persons with opioid use disorder in Massachusetts "reached 4.60% in 2015, nearly 4 times higher than current national prevalence estimates" (Barocas et al. 2018: 1679). One of the cornerstones to capture-recapture is its relative ease for replication studies. At both the local and federal level, studies can generate estimations of population densities in a wide array of geographical regions, including rural and remote locations which may lack the necessary resources to study the opioid population.

3.3 Conclusion

In order to generate a more complete understanding of the scope of the opioid epidemic, policy makers should consider accessing wider sources of data. The goal of this chapter was to provide the reader with a current overview of the wide array of data sources and methodologies that should be considered to further the knowledgebase of the opioid crisis. Notwithstanding, it is important to remember that all sources of data have some form of limitations and simply adding more 'bad' data only creates additional problems. Whether it is missing information such as in the case of attrition of death cases sent for MDI or a time lag for accessing prescription practices in a given jurisdiction, all sources of data will be incomplete in some manner. The additive function of including multiple sources of information allows for additional data "lenses" to be placed on the opioid crisis that may validate or contradict another data source. Carefully merging and analyzing the vast quantities of opioid-use data in a timely manner that ensures privacy laws are followed is a crucial next step developing a more complete evidence-base of needs and risks associated with the spectrum of opioid users.

References

Aliprantis, D., Fee, K., & Schweitzer, M. E. (2019). *Opioids and the labor market*. Cleveland, OH: Federal Reserve Bank of Cleveland (Working Paper No 18-7).

Allen, S. T., O'Rourke, A., White, R. H., Schneider, K. E., Kilkenny, M., & Sherman, S. G. (2019). Estimating the number of people who inject drugs in a rural county in Appalachia. *American Journal of Public Health, 109*(3), 445–450. https://doi.org/10.2105/AJPH.2018.304873.

Amram, O., Socías, E., Nosova, E., Kerr, T., Wood, E., DeBeck, K. … Milloy, M. J. (2019). Density of low-barrier opioid agonist clinics and risk of non-fatal overdose during a community-wide overdose crisis: A spatial analysis. *Spatial and Spatio-Temporal Epidemiology, 30*(0), 1–6. https://doi.org/10.1016/j.sste.2019.100288 .

Armenian, P., Vo, K. T., Barr-Walker, J., & Lynch, K. L. (2018). Fentanyl, fentanyl analogs and novel synthetic opioids: A comprehensive review. *Neuropharmacology, 134*, 121–132.

Axeen, S., Seabury, S. A., & Menchine, M. (2018). Emergency department contribution to the prescription opioid epidemic. *Annals of Emergency Medicine, 71*(6), 659–667. https://doi.org/10.1016/j.annemergmed.2017.12.007.

Babcock, C., Rockich-Winston, N., & Booth, C. (2017). Bringing naloxone to ground zero: Huntington, West Virginia. *Journal of the American Pharmacists Association, 57*(2), 9–10. https://doi.org/10.1016/j.japh.2016.09.006.

Barocas, J. A., White, L. F., Wang, J., Walley, A. Y., LaRochelle, M. R., Bernson, D. … Linas, B. P. (2018). Estimated prevalence of opioid use disorder in Massachusetts, 2011–2015: A capture–recapture analysis. *American Journal of Public Health, 108*(12), 1675–1681. https://doi.org/10.2105/ajph.2018.304673.

Been, F., Benaglia, L., Lucia, S., Gervasoni, J., Esseiva, P., & Delémont, O. (2015). Data triangulation in the context of opioids monitoring via wastewater analyses. *Drug and Alcohol Dependence, 151*(1), 203–210. https://doi.org/10.1016/j.drugalcdep.2015.03.022.

Bennett, A. S., Bell, A., Doe-Simkins, M., Elliott, L., Pouget, E., & Davis, C. (2018). From peers to lay bystanders: Findings from a decade of naloxone distribution in Pittsburgh, PA. *Journal of Psychoactive Drugs, 50*(3), 240–246. https://doi.org/10.1080/02791072.2018.1430409.

Boggess, S., & Bound, J. (1997). Did criminal activity increase during the 1980s? Comparisons across data sources. *Social Science Quarterly, 78*(3), 725–739.

Boslett, A. J., Denham, A., Hill, E. L., & Adams, M. C. (2019). Unclassified drug overdose deaths in the opioid crisis: Emerging patterns of inequity. *Journal of the American Medical Informatics Association, 0*(0), 1–11. https://doi.org/10.1093/jamia/ocz050.

Bouchard, M. (2007). A capture–recapture model to estimate the size of criminal populations and the risks of detection in a marijuana cultivation industry. *Journal of Quantitative Criminology, 23*(3), 221–241. https://doi.org/10.1007/s10940-007-9027-1.

Bronskill, J. (2018, August 14). Police chiefs call for stricter controls on pill presses to fight opioids. *The Canadian Press*. Retrieved from https://nationalpost.com.

Brooks Dollar, C. (2019). Criminalization and drug "Wars" or medicalization and health "Epidemics": How race, class, and neoliberal politics influence drug laws. *Critical Criminology, 27*(2), 305–327. https://doi.org/10.1007/s10612-018-9398-7.

Buchanich, J. M., Balmert, L. C., Williams, K. E., & Burke, D. S. (2018). The effect of incomplete death certificates on estimates of unintentional opioid-related overdose deaths in the united states, 1999–2015. *Public Health Reports, 133*(4), 423–431. https://doi.org/10.1177/0033354918774330.

Butler, M. M., Ancona, R. M., Beauchamp, G. A., Yamin, C. K., Winstanley, E. L., Hart, K. W. … Lindsell, C. J. (2016). Emergency department prescription opioids as an initial exposure preceding addiction. *Annals of Emergency Medicine, 68*(2), 202–208. https://doi.org/10.1016/j.annemergmed.2015.11.033.

Carpentier, C., Royuela, L., Montanari, L., & Davis, P. (2018). The global epidemiology of drug use in prison. In S. A. Kinner & J. D. Rich (Eds.), *Drug use in prisoners: Epidemiology,*

implications, and policy responses (pp. 17–41). New York, NY, US: Oxford University Press. https://doi.org/10.1093/med/9780199374847.003.0002.
Carter, J. G., Mohler, G., & Ray, B. (2019). Spatial concentration of opioid overdose deaths in Indianapolis: An application of the law of crime concentration at place to a public health epidemic. *Journal of Contemporary Criminal Justice, 35*(2), 161–185. https://doi.org/10.1177/1043986218803527.
Chandler, R. K., Fletcher, B. W., & Volkow, N. D. (2009). Treating drug abuse and addiction in the criminal justice system: Improving public health and safety. *Journal of the American Medical Association, 301*(2), 183–190. https://doi.org/10.1001/jama.2008.976.
Choi, S., Biello, K. B., Bazzi, A. R., & Drainoni, M. (2019). Age differences in emergency department utilization and repeat visits among patients with opioid use disorder at an urban safety-net hospital: A focus on young adults. *Drug and Alcohol Dependence, 200,* 14–18. https://doi.org/10.1016/j.drugalcdep.2019.02.030.
Christie, C., Baker, C., Cooper, R., Kennedy, P. J., Madras, B., & Bondi, P. (2017). *The president's commission on combating drug addiction and the opioid crisis.* Washington, D.C.: US Government Printing Office.
Ciccarone, D. (2019). The triple wave epidemic: Supply and demand drivers of the US opioid overdose crisis. *International Journal on Drug Policy, 0*(0), 1–6. https://doi.org/10.1016/j.drugpo.2019.01.010.
Cicero, T. J., Ellis, M. S., & Kasper, Z. A. (2017). Increased use of heroin as an initiating opioid of abuse. *Addictive Behaviors, 74,* 63–66. https://doi.org/10.1016/j.addbeh.2017.05.030.
Curtis, R., & Wendel, T. (2000). Toward the development of a typology of illegal drug markets. *Crime Prevention Studies, 11,* 121–152.
D'Onofrio, G., O'Connor, P. G., Pantalon, M. V., Chawarski, M. C., Busch, S. H., Owens, P. H. … Fiellin, D. A. (2015). Emergency department–initiated buprenorphine/naloxone treatment for opioid dependence: A randomized clinical trial. *Journal of the American Medical Association, 313*(16), 1636–1644. https://doi.org/10.1001/jama.2015.3474.
Dasgupta, N., Beletsky, L., & Ciccarone, D. (2018). Opioid crisis: No easy fix to its social and economic determinants. *American Journal of Public Health, 108*(2), 182–186. https://doi.org/10.2105/AJPH.2017.304187.
Davis, C. S., Ruiz, S., Glynn, P., Picariello, G., & Walley, A. Y. (2014). Expanded access to naloxone among firefighters, police officers, and emergency medical technicians in Massachusetts. *American Journal of Public Health, 104*(8), 7–9. https://doi.org/10.2105/AJPH.2014.302062.
Dowell, D., Haegerich, T. M., & Chou, R. (2016a). CDC guideline for prescribing opioids for chronic pain—United states, 2016. *Journal of the American Medical Association, 315*(15), 1624–1645. https://doi.org/10.1001/jama.2016.1464.
Dowell, D., Zhang, K., Noonan, R. K., & Hockenberry, J. M. (2016b). Mandatory provider review and pain clinic laws reduce the amounts of opioids prescribed and overdose death rates. *Health Affairs, 35*(10), 1876–1883. https://doi.org/10.1377/hlthaff.2016.0448.
Duber, H. C., Barata, I. A., Cioè-Peña, E., Liang, S. Y., Ketcham, E., Macias-Konstantopoulos, W. … Whiteside, L. K. (2018). Identification, management, and transition of care for patients with opioid use disorder in the emergency department. *Annals of Emergency Medicine, 72*(4), 420–431. https://doi.org/10.1016/j.annemergmed.2018.04.007.
Evoy, K. E., Hill, L. G., Groff, L., Mazin, L., Carlson, C. C., & Reveles, K. R. (2018). Naloxone accessibility without a prescriber encounter under standing orders at community pharmacy chains in Texas. *Journal of the American Medical Association, 320*(18), 1934–1937. https://doi.org/10.1001/jama.2018.15892.
Fischer, B., Vojtila, L., & Rehm, J. (2018). The 'fentanyl epidemic' in Canada–some cautionary observations focusing on opioid-related mortality. *Preventive Medicine, 107,* 109–113. https://doi.org/10.1016/j.ypmed.2017.11.001.
Frischer, M., Bloor, M., Finlay, A., Goldberg, D., Green, S., Haw, S. … Platt, S. (1991). A new method of estimating prevalence of injecting drug use in an urban population: Results from a Scottish city. *International Journal of Epidemiology, 20*(4), 997–1000.

Gilson, A. M., & Joranson, D. E. (2001). Controlled substances and pain management: Changes in knowledge and attitudes of state medical regulators. *Journal of Pain and Symptom Management, 21*(3), 227–237.

Giraudon, I., Lowitz, K., Dargan, P. I., Wood, D. M., & Dart, R. C. (2013). Prescription opioid abuse in the UK. *British Journal of Clinical Pharmacology, 76*(5), 823–824. https://doi.org/10.1111/bcp.12133.

Gladden, R. M. (2016). Fentanyl law enforcement submissions and increases in synthetic opioid—Involved overdose deaths—27 states, 2013–2014. *Morbidity and Mortality Weekly Report, 65* (33), 837–843. https://doi.org/10.15585/mmwr.mm6533a2.

Gupta, R., Shah, N. D., & Ross, J. S. (2016). The rising price of naloxone—Risks to efforts to stem overdose deaths. *New England Journal of Medicine, 375*(23), 2213–2215. https://doi.org/10.1056/NEJMp1609578.

Guy, J. G., Pasalic, E., & Zhang, K. (2018). Emergency department visits involving opioid overdoses, US, 2010–2014. *American Journal of Preventive Medicine, 54*(1), e39.

Hagemeier, N. E. (2018). Introduction to the opioid epidemic: The economic burden on the healthcare system and impact on quality of life. *The American Journal of Managed Care, 24* (10), S206.

Hamid, A. (1992). The developmental cycle of a drug epidemic: The cocaine smoking epidemic of 1981–1991. *Journal of Psychoactive Drugs, 24*(4), 337–348.

Han, B., Compton, W. M., Blanco, C., Crane, E., Lee, J., & Jones, C. M. (2017). Prescription opioid use, misuse, and use disorders in US adults: 2015 national survey on drug use and health. *Annals of Internal Medicine, 167*(5), 293–301. https://doi.org/10.7326/M17-0865.

Hedegaard, H., Warner, M., & Miniño, A. M. (2018). Drug overdose deaths in the united states, 1999–2017. *NCHS Data Brief, 329,* 1–8.

Hibdon, J., Telep, C. W., & Groff, E. R. (2017). The concentration and stability of drug activity in Seattle, Washington using police and emergency medical services data. *Journal of Quantitative Criminology, 33*(3), 497–517. https://doi.org/10.1007/s10940-016-9302-0.

Hingham, S., Horwitz, S., & Rich, S. (2019, July 16). *76 billion opioid pills: Newly released federal data unmasks the epidemic*. Retrieved from https://www.washingtonpost.com/.

Irvine, M. A., Kuo, M., Buxton, J., Balshaw, R., Otterstatter, M., Macdougall, L. … Tyndall, M. (2019). Modelling the combined impact of interventions in averting deaths during a synthetic-opioid overdose epidemic. *Addiction, 0*(0), 1–20. https://doi.org/10.1111/add.14664.

John, W. S., & Wu, L. (2019). Sex differences in the prevalence and correlates of emergency department utilization among adults with prescription opioid use disorder. *Substance Use and Misuse, 54*(7), 1178–1190. https://doi.org/10.1080/10826084.2019.1568495.

Johnson, B. D., Golub, A., & Fagan, J. (1995). Careers in crack, drug use, drug distribution, and nondrug criminality. *Crime & Delinquency, 41*(3), 275–295. https://doi.org/10.1177/0011128795041003001.

Jones, C. M., & McAninch, J. K. (2015). Emergency department visits and overdose deaths from combined use of opioids and benzodiazepines. *American Journal of Preventive Medicine, 49* (4), 493–501. https://doi.org/10.1016/j.amepre.2015.03.04.

Kelsall, D., & Bowes, M. J. (2016). No standards: Medicolegal investigation of deaths. *Canadian Medical Association Journal, 188*(3), 169. https://doi.org/10.1503/cmaj.160041.

Kilmer, B., Reuter, P., & Giommoni, L. (2015). What can be learned from cross-national comparisons of data on illegal drugs? *Crime and Justice, 44*(1), 227–296.

Kilwein, T. M., Wimbish, L. A., Gilbert, L., & Wambeam, R. A. (2019). Practices and concerns related to naloxone use among emergency medical service providers in a rural state: A mixed-method examination. *Preventive Medicine Reports, 14,* 1–6. https://doi.org/10.1016/j.pmedr.2019.100872.

Lambdin, B. H., Davis, C. S., Wheeler, E., Tueller, S., & Kral, A. H. (2018). Naloxone laws facilitate the establishment of overdose education and naloxone distribution programs in the United States. *Drug and Alcohol Dependence, 188,* 370–376. https://doi.org/10.1016/j.drugalcdep.2018.04.004 .

Lawton, Z. E., Traub, A., Fatigante, W. L., Mancias, J., O'Leary, A. E., Hall, S. E. … Mulligan, C. C. (2017). Analytical validation of a portable mass spectrometer featuring interchangeable, ambient ionization sources for high throughput forensic evidence screening. *Journal of the American Society for Mass Spectrometry, 28*(6), 1048–1059. https://doi.org/10.1007/s13361-016-1562-2.

Leong, M., Murnion, B., & Haber, P. S. (2009). Examination of opioid prescribing in Australia from 1992 to 2007. *Internal Medicine Journal, 39*(10), 676–681. https://doi.org/10.1111/j.1445-5994.2009.01982.x.

Lisa, B., & Jessica, H. (2018). Evidence synthesis-the opioid crisis in Canada: A national perspective. *Health Promotion and Chronic Disease Prevention in Canada: Research, Policy and Practice, 38*(6), 224–233. https://doi.org/10.24095/hpcdp.38.6.02.

Lovegrove, M. C., Dowell, D., Geller, A. I., Goring, S. K., Rose, K. O., Weidle, N. J., et al. (2019). US emergency department visits for acute harms from prescription opioid use, 2016–2017. *American Journal of Public Health, 109*(5), 784–791. https://doi.org/10.2105/AJPH.2019.305007.

MacDougall, L., Smolina, K., Otterstatter, M., Zhao, B., Chong, M., Godfrey, D. … Kendall, P. (2019). Development and characteristics of the provincial overdose cohort in British Columbia, Canada. *PloS One, 14*(1), 1–17. https://doi.org/10.1371/journal.pone.0210129.

Mars, S. G., Rosenblum, D., & Ciccarone, D. (2019). Illicit fentanyls in the opioid street market: Desired or imposed? *Addiction, 114*(5), 774–780. https://doi.org/10.1111/add.14474.

Marshall, J. R., Gassner, S. F., Anderson, C. L., Cooper, R. J., Lotfipour, S., & Chakravarthy, B. (2018). Socioeconomic and geographical disparities in prescription and illicit opioid-related overdose deaths in orange county, California, from 2010–2014. *Substance Abuse, 40*(1), 80–86. https://doi.org/10.1080/08897077.2018.1442899.

Mattson, C. L., O'Donnell, J., Kariisa, M., Seth, P., Scholl, L., & Gladden, R. M. (2018). Opportunities to prevent overdose deaths involving prescription and illicit opioids, 11 States, July 2016–June 2017. *Morbidity and Mortality Weekly Report, 67*(34), 945–951. https://doi.org/10.15585/mmwr.mm6734a2.

May, T., & Hough, M. (2004). Drug markets and distribution systems. *Addiction Research & Theory, 12*(6), 549–563. https://doi.org/10.1080/16066350412331323119.

McGowan, C. R., Harris, M., Platt, L., Hope, V., & Rhodes, T. (2018). Fentanyl self-testing outside supervised injection settings to prevent opioid overdose: Do we know enough to promote it? *International Journal of Drug Policy, 58,* 31–36. https://doi.org/10.1016/j.drugpo.2018.04.017.

Meldrum, M. L. (2003). A capsule history of pain management. *Journal of the American Medical Association, 290*(18), 2470–2475. https://doi.org/10.1001/jama.290.18.2470.

Melton, S. H., & Melton, S. T. (2019). Current state of the problem: Opioid overdose rates and deaths. *Current Treatment Options in Psychiatry, 6*(2), 164–177. https://doi.org/10.1007/s40501-019-00174-y.

Merino, R., Bowden, N., Katamneni, S., & Coustasse, A. (2019). The opioid epidemic in West Virginia. *The Health Care Manager, 38*(2), 187–195. https://doi.org/10.1097/hcm.0000000000000256.

Moe, J., Camargo, C. A., Jelinski, S., Erdelyi, S., Brubacher, J., & Rowe, B. H. (2018). Epidemiologic trends in substance and opioid misuse-related emergency department visits in Alberta: A cross-sectional time-series analysis. *Canadian Journal of Public Health, 109*(2), 164–173. https://doi.org/10.17269/s41997-018-0053-6.

Morrow, J. B., Ropero-Miller, J. D., Catlin, M. L., Winokur, A. D., Cadwallader, A. B., Staymates, J. L. … McCormick, M. M. (2019). The opioid epidemic: Moving toward an integrated, holistic analytical response. *Journal of Analytical Toxicology, 43*(1), 1–9. https://doi.org/10.1093/jat/bky049.

National Research Council. (2009). *Strengthening forensic science in the United States: A path forward.* Washington, D.C.: National Academies Press.

Ogbu, U. C., Lotfipour, S., & Chakravarthy, B. (2015). Polysubstance abuse: Alcohol, opioids and benzodiazepines require coordinated engagement by society, patients, and physicians. *Western Journal of Emergency Medicine, 16*(1), 76–79. https://doi.org/10.5811/westjem.2014.11.24720.

Paulozzi, L. J., Weisler, R. H., & Patkar, A. A. (2011). A national epidemic of unintentional prescription opioid overdose deaths how physicians can help control it. *The Journal of Clinical Psychiatry, 72*(5), 589–592. https://doi.org/10.4088/JCP.10com06560.

Peck, Y., Clough, A. R., Culshaw, P. N., & Liddell, M. J. (2019). Multi-drug cocktails: Impurities in commonly used illicit drugs seized by police in Queensland, Australia. *Drug and Alcohol Dependence, 201,* 49–57. https://doi.org/10.1016/j.drugalcdep.2019.03.019.

Pezalla, E. J., Rosen, D., Erensen, J. G., Haddox, J. D., & Mayne, T. J. (2017). Secular trends in opioid prescribing in the USA. *Journal of Pain Research, 10*(1), 383–387. https://doi.org/10.2147/JPR.S129553.

Plecas, D., McCormick, A. V., Levine, J., Neal, P., & Cohen, I. M. (2011). Evidence-based solution to information sharing between law enforcement agencies. *Policing: An International Journal of Police Strategies & Management, 34*(1), 120–134. https://doi.org/10.1108/13639511111106641.

Popper, N. (2019). *Dark web drug sellers dodge police crackdowns.* Retrieved from https://www.nytimes.com/2019/06/11/technology/online-dark-web-drug-markets.html.

Population DataBC. (2019). *About PopData.* Retrieved from https://www.popdata.bc.ca/aboutus.

Porter, J., & Jick, H. (1980). Addiction rare in patients treated with narcotics. *The New England Journal of Medicine, 302*(2), 123.

Postigo, C., de Alda, M., López, J., & Barceló, D. (2010). Drugs of abuse and their metabolites in the Ebro river basin: Occurrence in sewage and surface water, sewage treatment plants removal efficiency, and collective drug usage estimation. *Environment International, 36*(1), 75–84. https://doi.org/10.1016/j.envint.2009.10.004.

Rando, J., Broering, D., Olson, J. E., Marco, C., & Evans, S. B. (2015). Intranasal naloxone administration by police first responders is associated with decreased opioid overdose deaths. *The American Journal of Emergency Medicine, 33*(9), 1201–1204. https://doi.org/10.1016/j.ajem.2015.05.022.

Rees, D. I., Sabia, J. J., Argys, L. M., Latshaw, J., & Dave, D. (2019). With a little help from my friends: The effects of good Samaritan and naloxone access laws on opioid-related deaths. *The Journal of Law and Economics, 62*(1), 1–27. https://doi.org/10.1086/700703.

Rodwell, L., Ringland, C., & Bradford, D. (2010). *What do police data tell us about criminal methods of obtaining prescription drugs?* (No. 139). www.bocsar.nsw.gov.au. Bureau of Crime Statistics and Research New South Wales.

Rudd, R. A., Aleshire, N., Zibbell, J. E., & Matthew Gladden, R. (2016). Increases in drug and opioid overdose deaths—United states, 2000–2014. *American Journal of Transplantation, 16* (4), 1323–1327. https://doi.org/10.1111/ajt.13776.

Rummans, T. A., Burton, M. C., & Dawson, N. L. (2018). How good intentions contributed to bad outcomes: The opioid crisis. *Mayo Clinic Proceedings, 93*(3), 344–350. https://doi.org/10.1016/j.mayocp.2017.12.020.

Scheuermeyer, F. X., Grafstein, E., Buxton, J., Ahamad, K., Lysyshyn, M., DeVlaming, S. … Gustafson, R. (2019). Safety of a modified community trailer to manage patients with presumed fentanyl overdose. *Journal of Urban Health, 96*(1), 21–26. https://doi.org/10.1007/s11524-018-0321-z.

Schiff, D. M., Drainoni, M., Weinstein, Z. M., Chan, L., Bair-Merritt, M., & Rosenbloom, D. (2017). A police-led addiction treatment referral program in Gloucester, MA: Implementation and participants' experiences. *Journal of Substance Abuse Treatment, 82,* 41–47. https://doi.org/10.1016/j.jsat.2017.09.003.

Schneider, K. E., Park, J. N., Allen, S. T., Weir, B. W., & Sherman, S. G. (2019). Patterns of polysubstance use and overdose among people who inject drugs in Baltimore, Maryland: A latent class analysis. *Drug and Alcohol Dependence, 201,* 71–77. https://doi.org/10.1016/j.drugalcdep.2019.03.026.

Scholl, L., Seth, P., Kariisa, M., Wilson, N., & Baldwin, G. (2019). Drug and opioid-involved overdose deaths—United states, 2013–2017. *Morbidity and Mortality Weekly Report, 67*(51 & 52), 1–9.

Skinner, J., Carter, L., & Haxton, C. (2009). Case management of patients who frequently present to a Scottish emergency department. *Emergency Medicine Journal, 26*(2), 103–105. https://doi.org/10.1136/emj.2008.063081.

Toblin, R. L., Quartana, P. J., Riviere, L. A., Walper, K. C., & Hoge, C. W. (2014). Chronic pain and opioid use in US soldiers after combat deployment. *JAMA Internal Medicine, 174*(8), 1400–1401. https://doi.org/10.1001/jamainternmed.2014.2726.

Tyndall, M. (2018). An emergency response to the opioid overdose crisis in Canada: A regulated opioid distribution program. *Canadian Medical Association Journal, 190*(2), E36.

van Nuijs, A. L., Castiglioni, S., Tarcomnicu, I., Postigo, C., de Alda, M. L., Neels, H. … Covaci, A. (2011). Illicit drug consumption estimations derived from wastewater analysis: A critical review. *Science of the Total Environment, 409*(19), 3564–3577. https://doi.org/10.1016/j.scitotenv.2010.05.030.

Vivolo-Kantor, A. M., Seth, P., Gladden, R. M., Mattson, C. L., Baldwin, G. T., Kite-Powell, A., et al. (2018). Trends in emergency department visits for suspected opioid overdoses—United states, July 2016–September 2017. *Morbidity and Mortality Weekly Report, 67*(9), 279–285. https://doi.org/10.15585/mmwr.mm6709e1.

Wall, R., Rehm, J., Fischer, B., Gliksman, L., Stewart, J., Medved, W., et al. (2000). Social costs of untreated opioid dependence. *Journal of Urban Health, 77*(4), 688–722. https://doi.org/10.1007/bf02344032.

White, H. R., & Gorman, D. M. (2000). Dynamics of the drug-crime relationship. *Criminal Justice, 1*(15), 1–218.

Winkelman, T. N., Chang, V. W., & Binswanger, I. A. (2018). Health, polysubstance use, and criminal justice involvement among adults with varying levels of opioid use. *JAMA Network Open, 1*(3), 1–12. https://doi.org/10.1001/jamanetworkopen.2018.0558.

Wood, E., Spittal, P. M., Small, W., Kerr, T., Li, K., Hogg, R. S. … Schechter, M. T. (2004). Displacement of Canada's largest public illicit drug market in response to a police crackdown. *Canadian Medical Association Journal, 170*(10), 1551–1556. https://doi.org/10.1503/cmaj.1031928.

Yokell, M. A., Delgado, M. K., Zaller, N. D., Wang, N. E., McGowan, S. K., & Green, T. C. (2014). Presentation of prescription and nonprescription opioid overdoses to US emergency departments. *JAMA Internal Medicine, 174*(12), 2034–2037. https://doi.org/10.1001/jamainternmed.2014.5413.

Part II
Geography of Crime

Chapter 4
Crime Hot Spots, Crime Corridors and the Journey to Crime: An Expanded Theoretical Model of the Generation of Crime Concentrations

Paul J. Brantingham, Patricia L. Brantingham, Justin Song and Valerie Spicer

4.1 The Fact of Hot Spots

The fact of hot spots—spatial and temporal concentrations of crime in the aggregate—has become one of the most important contributions of environmental criminology both to contemporary criminological research and to criminal justice practice (Lee et al. 2017; Weisburd 2015; Sherman and Weisburd 1995; Weisburd et al. 1993; Sherman et al. 1989). Spatial and temporal crime concentrations have been found in the crime data of many different countries: Brazil, Canada, China, England, India, Israel, the Netherlands, Sweden, Trinidad and Tobago, and the United States, among others. It has served as a springboard to explorations of the concentrations in time and space of crimes as diverse as car theft (Fleming et al. 1994; Hesseling 1995), gang violence (Block and Block 1993), burglary (Hirschfield et al. 1995; Bennett 1995), liquor and drugs related crimes (Block and Block 1995; Block 1990; Roncek and Maier 1991), robbery (Hipp and Young-An 2019); transit related crimes (Block and Davis 1996; Buckley 1996), murder (Coburn 1988; Bullock 1955); domestic violence (Verma et al. 1994); and, terrorism (Perry 2019). The fact of hot spots of crime has also served as the starting point for identifying and attacking drug markets (Edmunds et al. 1996) and as a tool both for mounting both police crackdowns (Buerger et al. 1995; Sherman and

P. J. Brantingham (✉) · P. L. Brantingham · J. Song · V. Spicer
Simon Fraser University, Burnaby, Canada
e-mail: branting@sfu.ca

P. L. Brantingham
e-mail: pbrantin@sfu.ca

J. Song
e-mail: jdsong@sfu.ca

V. Spicer
e-mail: vspicer@sfu.ca

K. M. Lersch and J. Chakraborty (eds.), *Geographies of Behavioural Health, Crime, and Disorder*, GeoJournal Library 126,
https://doi.org/10.1007/978-3-030-33467-3_4

Weisburd 1995) and for targeting crime prevention resources (Bennett 1995; Hesseling 1995; Barclay et al. 1996). The potential for using hot spots for targeting effective primary, secondary and tertiary crime prevention actions of all sorts seems to us to be enormous. With limited exceptions (e.g., Block and Block 1995: 117; Langworthy and LeBeau 1992a, b; Eck 1996) however, little work appears to have been done on the development of a general theory of the formation of hot spots of crime in time and space. David Weisburd's theoretical work on the law of crime concentration has advanced some important arguments on the implications of hot spots for criminal justice practice without addressing why hot spots form at particular places and at particular times (see, e.g., Weisburd 2015; Weisburd et al. 1993)

4.1.1 Crime Corridors

Recent research has demonstrated that thinking about crime concentration should be expanded from the idea of hot spots to also include the phenomena of crime corridors—extended corridors of elevated crime levels that run along streets through cities. Such corridors have been demonstrated in studies of the crime patterns and concentrations in Seattle (Weisburd et al. 2012), Vancouver (Curman et al. 2015) and Albany, New York (Wheeler et al. 2016). Figure 4.1 shows the crime concentrations in a major Canadian city during the mid-2000s using one aspect of street profile analysis (Spicer et al. 2016). Both *hot spots* (large numbers of crime occurring in close spatial proximity) and *crime corridors* (sets of crime clusters running along particular roads or paths) are visible. Three layers of information are utilized: a road network, an underlying pattern of land uses keyed in relatively pale colors; and a top layer displaying the location of recorded criminal events in this city as vertical spikes. Increasing crime counts range from no crime spikes to low counts in green to middling counts in yellow to higher counts in orange to highest counts in red.

4.1.2 Burning Times: Concentration of Crimes in Time

The variance in the occurrence of crime at different times has long been a staple of criminology. Crime volumes vary seasonally, weekly, daily and hourly. Both crime hot spots and crime corridors have been shown to be persistent over long periods of time: the Seattle and Vancouver studies both identified crime concentrations that were stable over more than a decade and a half. An additional issue is the extent to which crime concentrations which are stable over the long term nevertheless fluctuate over shorter time periods: a robbery hot spot might consistently appear at the same spatial location over the course of a year, but might only actually experience crimes between 9:00 p.m. and 1:00 a.m., for instance (see, e.g., Hipp and

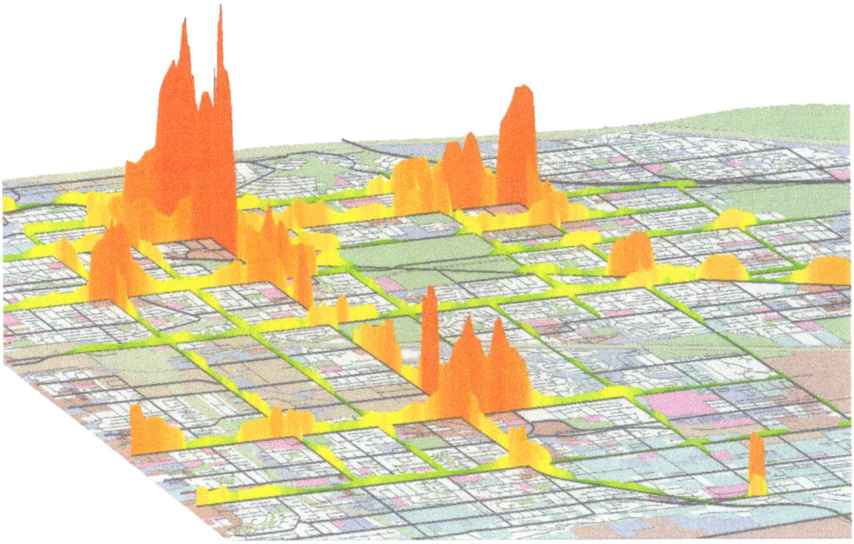

Fig. 4.1 Crime hot spots and crime corridors in a large Canadian city

Young-An 2019; Johnson et al. 2008). Figure 4.2 shows the variance in the structure—the volume and spatial concentration of crimes—of a persistent crime hot spot in Vancouver over different periods of the day:

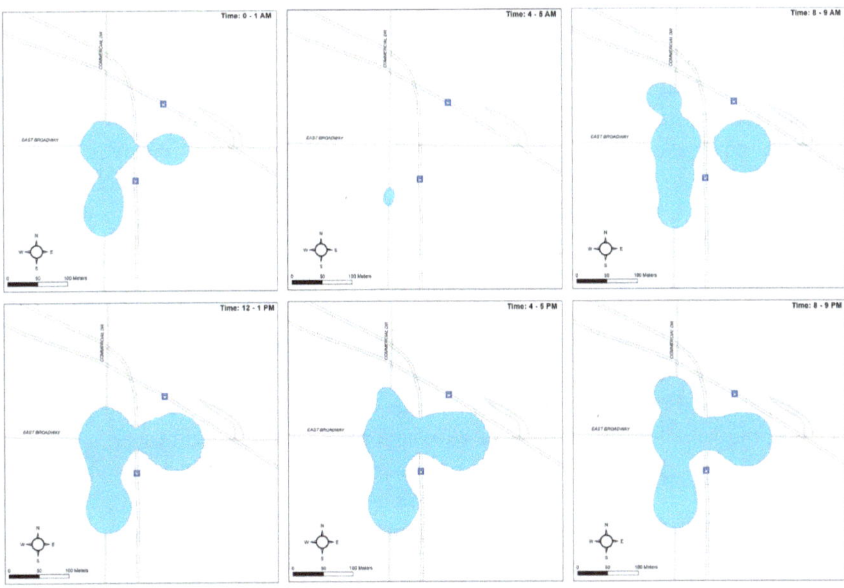

Fig. 4.2 Variation in crime patterns at a persistent hot spot during different times of the day

Using crime pattern theory, the Brantinghams proposed a theory of crime hot spot formation to account for why criminal events concentrate in particular places and times (Brantingham and Brantingham 1999) focusing on the factors that structure criminal opportunities and events and the major components of the lived environment. This theoretical model has been shown to provide an effective tool for predicting the empirical patterns in the formation crime concentrations (Deryol et al. 2016) but can be improved by further attention to some of its component ideas. We believe that our original model can be enhanced by attention to the theory of offender target search in its relation to key principles of Crime Pattern Theory.

4.2 A Theory of Hot Spot Formation

The formation of hot spots and burning times can sometimes be explained or predicted fairly simply with straightforward building blocks drawn from environmental criminology where crimes are seen as the result of multi-staged decisions (both conscious and unconscious) that depend on the surrounding environment in interaction with the potential offender's motivation. Sometimes the explanation for hot spot formation will require careful thought and inquiry. We believe that a useful approach is to think in terms of the structural elements of pattern theory (Brantingham and Brantingham 1993a) in conjunction with the theory of target search (Brantingham and Brantingham 2013) and to consider them in terms of conceptual layers setting out crime potentials in time and space. Each layer has a meaning and is a reflection of factors influencing where crimes occur. It might be easier to think of layers as overlays placed on a projector where part of the overlay is transparent, part opaque, and other parts with varying levels of opacity. Layers can then be "piled" one on top of another and the crime potentials for all levels summed for any given location in space time. The placing of one layer on another, using this analogue, changes the final degree of opacity. Some areas will be clear, others will allow some light through. Others still will allow little or no light through. The dark areas represent the areas where crime concentration is expected.

Hot spots form at the confluence of high crime potentials from some multiplicity of predisposing environmental conditions and activities operating at different elemental levels. These conditions include the residential and activity locations for predisposed offender populations, the residential and activity locations of vulnerable populations, the broader residential and activity structures of a city, the mix of activity types and land uses, the modes of transport and the structure of the transport network, the actual transportation flows of people in the city's timescape influence what becomes a crime generator or crime attractor. Figure 4.3 illustrates this idea in the abstract.

Figure 4.4 illustrates this idea more concretely by conceptualizing the building blocks of a hot spot in terms of levels or layers of crime potential. By overlaying these crime potential layers and looking down through the layers, looking for areas of overlap, we can see places where hot spots are most likely to form. In Fig. 4.4,

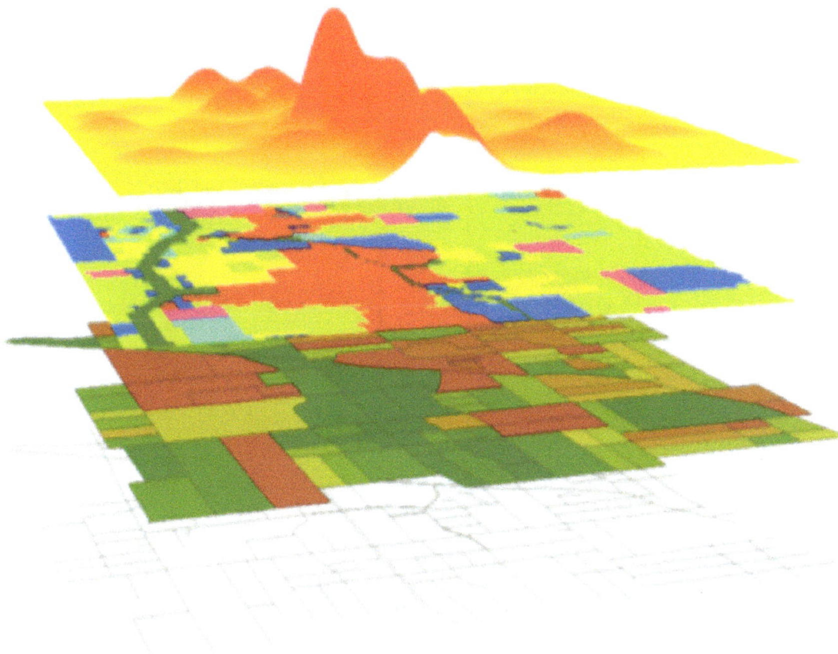

Fig. 4.3 Layers of crime potential

the first layer of the map identifies a low Social Efficacy residential area. Such areas often include the residences of a disproportionate number occasional and repeat offenders.

The second layer identifies the major traffic arteries. As discussed below, such roads are known to structure the search for crime sites within any given neighborhood. These are the primary travel and crime target routes for neighborhood "insiders" and for "outsiders" passing through as well.

Layer 3 identifies the major pedestrian stopping points in the area. In this case we posit a school and a cluster of shops. Both types of land uses, as discussed below, are known to be crime generators.

The fourth panel in Fig. 4.4 shows a composite of the three crime potential layers. As areas of the three layers overlap, they appear darker. The darkest areas represent the places where crime hot spots are most likely to form.

Viewing these layers together makes it possible to see the natural patterns of movement for the people who use the area, the location of potential offenders and potential targets. This provides a reasonable initial explanation for a concentration or clustering of crimes. We provide an example of this model, using data from Vancouver, later in this paper. First, however, we think it useful to turn to a more detailed discussion of the elements of these crime potential layers.

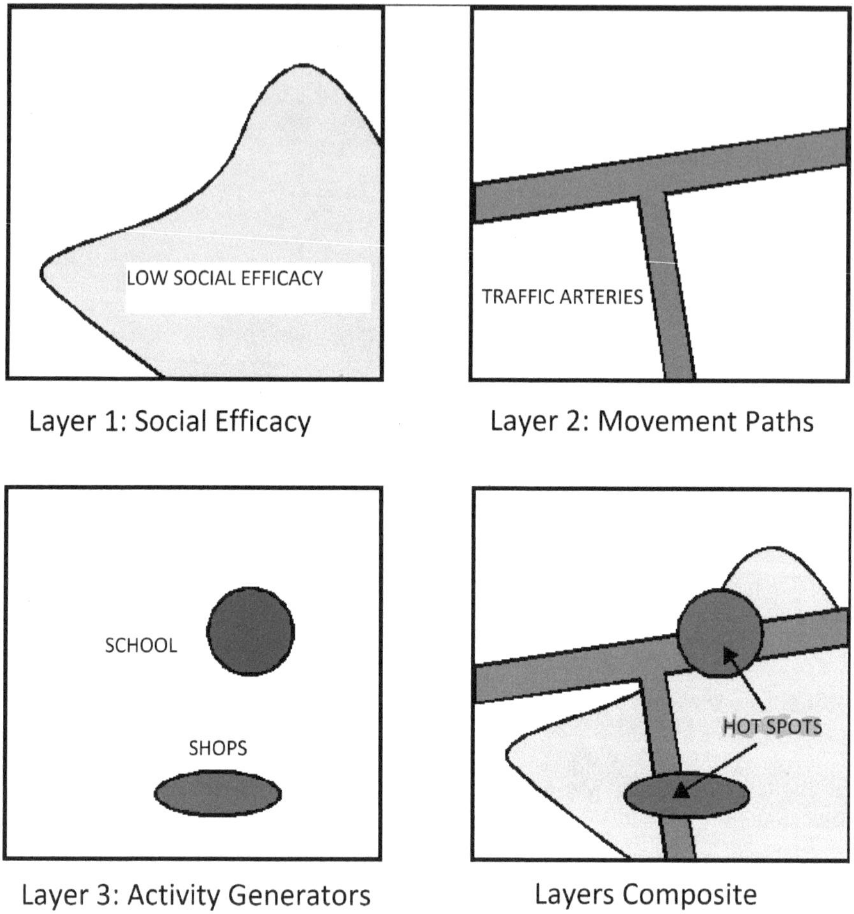

Fig. 4.4 Crime potential layers contributing to hotspot creation: simplified model

We find it helpful to describe these levels or layers of crime potential as the *environmental backcloth*, in general, with a more detailed description of:

- Concentrations of criminal residences;
- Concentrations of criminal targets;
- Normal movement patterns,
- The location of potential crime generators,
- The location of potential crime attractors,
- The structure of the path network, and
- Ecological labels.

4.2.1 The Environmental Backcloth

Events transpire at an immediate foreground site and situation that is enmeshed with a backcloth composed of interactions between the physical, social, legal, cultural, economic and temporal environments[1] functioning jointly and holistically. Elements of the backcloth are interconnected and never static. Change is a constant condition of the backcloth, but the types of changes, degrees of change and rates of change are varied and are extremely important. LeBeau's research exploring the importance to crime of changes in the structure of Charlotte, North Carolina, over time and space provides visual and statistical images of the non-static nature of behavior (e.g., LeBeau 1995).

Although the backcloth[2] is a holistic concept, it may be decomposed into different dimensions for analytic purposes. It can be convenient to think in terms of a structural backcloth and an activity backcloth. The **structural backcloth** is composed of relatively slowly changing elements such as laws, social norms, class structures, the division of labor, the physical layout of the built environment, the local topography, the local climate and so forth. In developing their Risk Terrain Modeling tools, Caplan and Kennedy and their associates have developed a practical approach to modeling parts of the structural backcloth (e.g., Caplan et al. 2011, 2013). The **activity backcloth** is composed of routines and adventures and is shaped by mobility and awareness factors that are tied to personality, age, social status, income, education and a variety of other social and psychological characteristics, as well as to positioning in physical space-time.

In thinking about the backcloth underlying hot spot formation, there are at least two broad groupings of issues that need to be taken into account overtly. These groupings of issues form two operational layers in a theory of hot spots. First, we need to consider a layer that draws on work in the long tradition of the cartographers and ecologists of crime and tells us about relatively fixed concentrations of criminal residences. Second, we need to think about the concentration of criminal targets.

4.2.1.1 Criminal Residence Concentration

The study of crime concentration began with studies of the concentration of criminal residences rather than the study of criminal events. The fact of such criminal neighborhoods has been long established in the work of both Mayhew and Booth in the 19th century, in the work of Burgess (1925a, b) and Shaw and McKay

---

[1]Obviously, given our conceptualization of the backcloth, any enumeration of this sort is inadequate and is provided merely as a rhetorical convenience.

[2]Operationalized, the backcloth often looks much like the idea of "context" advanced by recent works in human ecology, but is the term we prefer because it carries a dynamic, changing meaning with it. Context, on the other hand, is seen by some as more a stationary control to limit variability.

(1942), Morris (1958), Baldwin and Bottoms (1976) and many others in the 20th century. Indeed, the assumption of concentration of criminal neighborhoods is fundamental to much theory and research on the social origins of criminality, particularly in the social disorganization/social efficacy tradition.

The distribution of concentrations of criminal residence creates one level of crime potential. Most offenders commit most their crimes close to home. A crime hot spot can form on the basis of a concentration of criminal residences (see, e.g., Bennett 1995; Rhodes and Conly 1991; Costanzo et al. 1986; Capone and Nichols 1976; Pyle 1974; Menting 2018).

When offenders commit offences away from home these offences distribute in the direction of some additional important life node—work, school, a downtown entertainment district, an illegal drug market or the shop of a receiver of stolen property. The directional distortion in such crime distributions sets up a potential confluence between the target searching fields of many offenders (Rengert 1994; Weisburd et al. 1994; Langworthy and LeBeau 1992a, b; Rengert and Wasilchick 1985; Brantingham and Brantingham 1981; Baldwin and Bottoms 1976; Pyle 1974).

4.2.1.2 Ecological Theories

Ecological predictions of criminal residence locations were first made as part of a broader set of studies of competition for social space in the growing cities of the United States during the first third of the 20th century. Burgess' model of urban form (1925a) defined urban structure in terms of concentric zones of social use that were shaped by economic values and travel times defined in relation to a city's economic activity center. Taking into account the impact of building life cycles under conditions of population growth, Burgess predicted the development of an impoverished transitional zone at the outer edge of the central business district, and also predicted similar, less intense transitional zones surrounding subsidiary business districts. Under conditions of urban growth these transitional areas become residential collectors of the city's outcasts: economic immigrants; proscribed minorities; paupers and criminals.

The Burgess model[3] predicts concentrations of criminal residence in locations arrayed around city centers. Such areas could be identified independently of crime data on the basis of typical urban planning data such as the ratio of older housing stock to new business uses or the structure of the transport and street networks; and on the basis of typical census data such as rate of residential turnover, median income, and ethnic mix. Such concentrations have been found in most North American studies (see, Brantingham and Brantingham 1984 for a summary), and

[3]In our view, Burgess' model is more complex and substantially more powerful than the simplified version familiar to criminologists through the work of such disciples as Shaw (1929), Shaw and McKay (1942) or Schmid (1960a, b).

also appear in European studies despite the more substantial governmental controls over housing and urban development (Baldwin and Bottoms 1976; Bottoms and Xanthos 1981; Wikstrom 1991). Moreover, the ecological model predicts long term stability in the location of such concentrations, keyed to the life cycle of residential construction.

4.2.1.3 Housing Competition Theories

Sir Anthony Bottoms (see, e.g., Bottoms and Xanthos 1981; Bottoms and Wiles 1986) has led the way into consideration of the more complicated distributions of criminal residences found in cities in which governments play a major role in the housing market. Government housing allocation policies and practices (often operating in concert with tenant choice) create concentrations of criminal residence in locations different from those predicted by traditional criminal ecology. Competition for housing occurs through the manipulation of bureaucratic allocation rules rather than purely through spending on rent or mortgage payments, but still results in concentrations of urban outcasts. Such concentrations can be discerned from justice system data and can, in principle, be predicted from other social information (Wikstrom 1991).

4.2.1.4 Target Concentration

Targets of crime are as important to the development of hot spots as criminal residences. Although some sorts of targets are approaching ubiquity in contemporary cities—valuable electronic goods, for instance—most types of crime targets are dispersed unevenly across space and time. Many kinds of crime targets are concentrated by land uses and movement patterns. Some types of land uses provide substantial concentrations of targets. Shopping malls, for instance, provide concentrations of goods exposed to shoplifting; concentrations of unattended automobiles that can be broken into, stolen or criminally damaged; clusters of loitering niches that can accommodate either rowdy teenagers or discreet drug dealers; and concentrations of female shoppers who could be pursued by sexual deviants. Entertainment districts create nighttime concentrations of relaxed and often inebriated people. Some types of transit systems and some types of travel paths concentrate targets at predictable times. The routine activities of everyday life create concentrations of targets at predictable places at predictable times (Felson 1994).

4.2.1.5 Land Use Theories

Potential targets for crime are not ubiquitously distributed. Land uses concentrate in particular locations both for economic reasons and because of land use controls. Land uses and their locations change over time. Over the past half-century, the markets in many urban areas have changed from central agglomerations of street vendors and small shops to suburban mega malls and "big box" shopping areas. Many cities are now trying to re-introduce market stall areas as part of a gentrification and re-construction of city center neighborhoods. Housing patterns have evolved from cottages to modernist blocks of suites to the currently fashionable post-modern "new urbanism" style. Social services have moved from the small, local office to the large, centralized locations and are currently moving back to what is called a "human" scale.

These changes in urban form and style over time are tied very closely to normative theories about how cities *should* function and to explanatory theories about how cities actually grow and change. With some exceptions, these theories are imbedded within an understanding that cities, places within cities, and even areas within individual buildings, form a type of hierarchy with concentrations of different activities in different areas at different levels in the hierarchy. In normative theories about how the city should function, this hierarchy is often seen as a clearly defined ordering with, for example, one paramount city center, four regional shopping centres arrayed in each quadrant around the city center, and a series of smaller local area centres radiating out from the regional centres. In approaches that explore how cities really grow, the depiction of city structure becomes more complex and is seen to be dependent on many factors ranging from the topographical to the sets of organizational and governmental constraints and encouragements. To our knowledge, the Sheffield studies initiated by Baldwin and Bottoms (1976) remains the best continuing examination of the interplay of topography (Sheffield's intense mix sharp escarpments and deep valleys) and strong governmental housing policies and social processes in shaping the crime patterns of an urban complex (e.g., Bottoms and Xanthos 1981; Bottoms and Wiles 1986; Bottoms 1994). To a lesser degree this interplay has also been explored in Wikstrom's Stockholm studies (1985, 1991) and in the classic Chicago School studies (Shaw and McKay 1942).

The non-random distribution of land uses in cities creates both concentrations of crime targets and many areas and times containing few targets. Entertainment areas, particularly those with clusters of drinking establishments; shopping malls; and transit routes all produce concentrations of people where assaults are more likely (entertainment areas—see, e.g., Verma 1996; Block and Block 1995; Wikstrom 1991; Roncek and Maier 1991; Engstad 1975; Bullock 1955); places for shop lifting, theft from auto, theft of auto and disputes between juvenile groups (shopping malls, see, e.g., Brantingham et al. 1990); and concentrations of people where theft, robbery and assault can easily occur (major transit stops, see, e.g., Buckley 1996; Block and Davis 1996; Brantingham et al. 1991).

4.2.1.6 Routine Activity Theories

Routine activity theories predict that the routine rhythms of daily life will create concentrations of targets. The routines of work concentrate people and automobiles in different parts of the city at different times of the day. The routines of shopping, of work, and of recreation create concentrations of targets at malls, in city center parking garages, in entertainment districts at different times of the day and on different days of the week. These routines create the potential for hot spot formation.

4.2.1.7 The Intersection of Criminal Residence Residential and Crime Target Concentrations

Crime Pattern Theory suggests that in the aggregate, a metropolitan region's crime hot spots should be spatially related to but not completely congruent with concentrations of criminals' residences. Crime hot spots should also be related to major activity nodes near offender residence neighborhoods. Figure 4.5 illustrates this point with data from suburban Vancouver during the mid-2000s. Figure 4.5a shows the concentrations of known offender residences. Figure 4.5b shows the known crime hot spots. Figure 4.5c overlays the two maps, showing the congruence between concentrations of criminal residences and known hot spots of crime. The patterns are clearly related but not perfectly congruent.

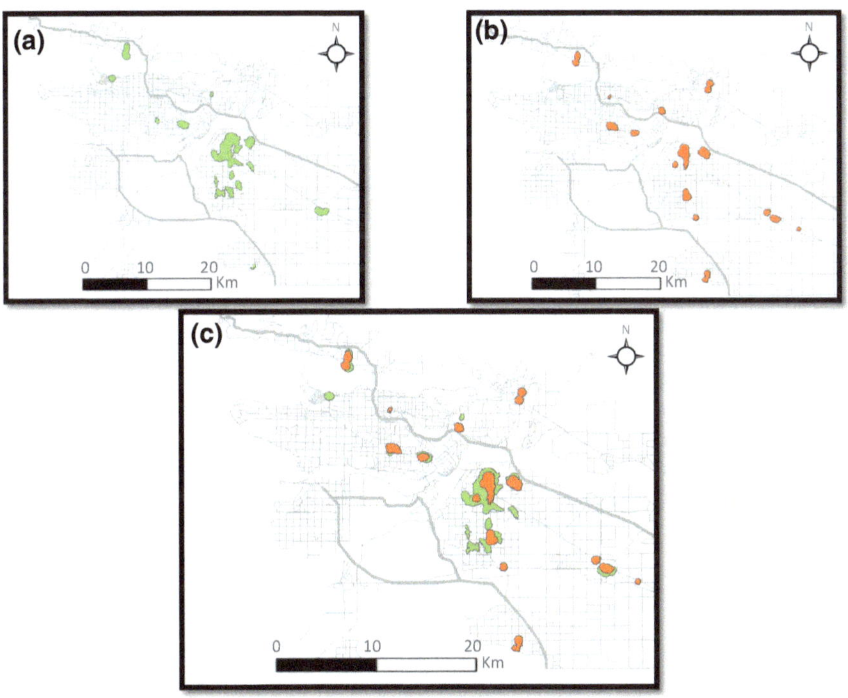

Fig. 4.5 Concentrations of criminal residences and crimes

4.2.2 Movement Patterns

Movement is a critical component in hot spot formation. The modes of transport, the rhythms of movement, the volumes of movement and the ease of flow along different transportation paths all create concentrations of offenders and targets at predictable times and places (Burgess 1925a; Brantingham et al. 1991; Angel 1968; Lowe and Moryadas 1975; Reid et al. 2014). Buckley (1996) has shown how transit stations in Vancouver create intense hot spots accounting for major portions of that city's crime while Block and Davis (1996) have shown how some crime problems radiate from the elevated train stations in Chicago. Brantingham and Brantingham (1995a) have shown how intersecting transit nodes concentrate crime in Burnaby, a principal suburb of Vancouver. A number of scholars have shown how the spatial distribution crimes as diverse as residential burglary (Fink 1969; Maguire 1982) and serial murder (e.g., Rossmo 1994) can be shaped by the location of motor way exits. Wilcox (1973) demonstrated that robbery is distributed according to the distribution of arterial and collector roads in Oakland, California. The distribution of thefts and car thefts in metropolitan Vancouver have been shown to be a function of road network connectivity (Beavon et al. 1994; Weigman and Hu 1992). White (1990) has shown that American residential burglary rates are a function of the extent to which the roads and lane ways of a neighborhood make it permeable to external traffic.

This body of work emphasizes the criminological importance of policy and practice in urban planning. Development decisions taken by city councils, town planning units, traffic engineering departments, rapid transit authorities and similar governmental bodies charged with matters usually thought to be unrelated to crime in fact have substantial impact on crime patterns. Criminologists need to find better ways of communicating this information to these governmental bodies and working cooperatively in a policy arena they do not typically enter. Plotting the locations and interconnections of transit nodes and other channels of movement such as restricted access motor ways, traffic arterial roads, and even major pedestrian foot paths in conjunction with analysis of road network ease-of-flow measures[4] should make it possible for criminologists to anticipate the development of many crime hot spots and to suggest ways to cool those hot spots without appreciable displacement effects. An expanded set of studies conducted in a growing number of cities should make it possible for criminologists to develop a calibrated weighting scale that could be used to assess how the intersection of different movement patterns at any specific location increases that location's crime potential.

[4]Appropriate measures are likely to be drawn from graph theory and include a location's associated number, its accessibility index, a *beta* index of connectivity across the entire network, and a location's *gamma* index of connectedness. See, Brantingham and Brantingham (1984: 240–243).

4.2.2.1 Target Searches and Journeys to Crime

The offender's search for criminal targets or victims can be seen from the perspective movement away from some activity base (such as home or a friend's house or a work site) to the crime site—a journey to crime which may or may not result in spatial or temporal concentrations of crime. We can identify four different kinds of journeys to crime by offenders (Brantingham and Brantingham 2013): proximity events, opportunistic discoveries; purposive searches and information-led searches.

4.2.2.2 Proximity Events

Proximity events require little or no target search by the offender. The victim or target is in the immediate presence or vicinity of the offender at the moment that some provocation or temptation triggers the criminal action (Brantingham and Brantingham 1978, 1984). Common assaults and domestic homicides are exemplars of provocation-driven proximity events, but robbery also happens in this way (Feeney 1986; Gabor et al. 1987; Wright and Decker 1997). Even when there is a delay between provocation and criminal attack, the identity and location of the target is known to the offender from the interaction constituting the provocation. Temptation-driven proximity exemplars could include employee pilfering of office supplies or shop inventory and many forms of embezzlement.

Proximity events are likely to exhibit limited spatial concentration. Such concentrations of proximity events as do occur are likely to be found in socially disadvantaged neighborhoods where the strains and stresses of daily life give rise to provocations and temptations. Proximity events may well show temporal concentrations keyed to personal interaction times or office times.

4.2.2.3 Opportunistic Discoveries

A large proportion of all criminal events are purely opportunistic in the sense that the offender was engaged in some non-criminal activity away from home, discovered an opportunity for crime that was too good to resist during the course of that activity, and acted on the opportunity—either immediately or relatively soon thereafter. Bruce Jacobs (2010) has described this process as *serendipity*. No crime was intended and no target search occurred. As Marcus Felson and Ronald Clarke have argued, sometimes opportunity makes the crime (1998).

Opportunistic crimes can be expected to concentrate in those neighborhoods in which known criminals reside. They will also concentrate in and around crime generators—high activity points such as transit stations, schools, sports stadiums, entertainment districts, shopping centers, and along the arterial travel paths between residential neighborhoods and activity centers.

4.2.2.4 Purposive Target Searches

Purposive target searches involve intending offenders who have a particular type of crime in mind but do not have a specific target already chosen. A purposive search unfolds as a multi-staged journey and decision process in which the offender first selects a general target area based on distance from the offender's starting point, directional relation to some major aggregate activity node, physical accessibility, social accessibility and some presumed supply of targets for the type of crime being contemplated (Brantingham and Brantingham 1978; Cromwell et al. 1991; Cornish 1994; Hakim et al. 2001; Boivin and D'Elia 2017). To some extent this multi-staged model is now seen as roughly akin to optimal foraging theory as it is understood in ecology and anthropology (Brantingham 2006; Bernasco 2009; Johnson et al. 2009).

Purposive target search may keep the offender in his or her home neighborhood; or it may take the offender to some other, very similar neighborhood with which the offender is familiar; or it may take the offender to some crime attractor—a high aggregate activity point with a presumed concentration of potential targets. In the aggregate, purposive target searches are likely to produce crime concentrations in neighborhoods with high offender residency, in similar neighborhoods arrayed along major pathways to activity nodes and at some attractor nodes.

4.2.2.5 Information-Led Target Searches

Some crime trips, particularly those undertaken by persistent professional criminals, are organized around information about the location of specific types of targets (for instance, banks or jewelry stores) or about a specific space-time location of a very specific target (a drug shipment for hi-jacking; an armored car moving cash to refill ATM's; a hired murderer's intended victim; a wealthy home whose occupants are away on a Caribbean cruise). Information-led crimes will almost always have unique space-time characteristics and will not, except coincidentally, be related to crime hot spots.

This information about the criminogenic potential of human movement and mobility patterns and the character of the journey to crime can, we believe, be combined with what is known about the criminogenic potential of concentrations of land use, the spatial segregation of social activity, the polarization of different socio-economic groups within different urban areas, the patterns of routine activities associated with different life styles and site specific design choices so as to make it possible for criminologists to identify crime generators and predict the formation of crime hot spots.

4.2.2.6 Crime Generators

Crime generators are specific sites or land uses or locales to which large numbers of people are attracted for reasons unrelated to crime. Typical examples might include shopping precincts; shopping malls; entertainment districts; office districts; and large housing complexes or estates. Specific individual land uses, businesses or activity destinations can also become crime generators, provided they large volumes of people. Examples might include large schools, sports stadiums, or theme parks such as Disneyland.

As we have already argued, major travel nodes, where many different travel paths and transit modes converge or intersect, can form crime generators. Bus interchanges, transit system stops, massive 'park and ride' parking lots can all become crime generators because of the volumes of people that pass through them. The heavily traveled paths *between* activity sites can also form crime generators as people traveling along them on legitimate business notice opportunities for crime or become exposed to resident criminals.

Crime generators produce crime by creating particular times and places that provide appropriate concentrations of people and other targets (Frank et al. 2011; Angel 1968; Wilcox 1973) in settings that are conducive to particular types of criminal acts. Mixed among the people gathered at crime generator locations are potential offenders who, although they did not travel to the area with the explicit intent of doing a crime, happen to notice and exploit those criminal opportunities presented by the generator location.[5]

The dynamics of crime at generator locations suggest that hot spots for different types of crime may occur in spatially congruent locations or may occur in different locations and that some persistent crime hot spots may experience crimes only during certain different times when population and target densities and backcloth conditions meet offender crime template requirements (Kinney et al. 2008; Haberman 2017; Demeau and Parent 2018; Hipp and Young-An 2019; Boivin and Nogueira de Melo 2019).

4.2.2.7 Crime Attractors

Crime attractors are particular places, areas, neighborhoods, or districts which create well known criminal opportunities to which strongly motivated, intending criminal offenders are attracted because of the known opportunities for particular types of crime. Examples might include bar districts; drug markets; large shopping malls, particularly those near major public transit exchanges; large, insecure parking lots in business or commercial areas.

[5]This sometimes happens immediately following the discovery of the opportunity, but not always. Offenders state that they often notice some opportunity which they remember and return to exploit at a later, more convenient or less risky time.

Crimes in such locations are often committed by area outsiders. Strongly motivated offenders will travel relatively long distances in search of a target (e.g., Menting 2018; Boivin and D'Elia 2017; Frank et al. 2011; Capone and Nichols 1976). When insiders commit crimes in such areas, they may have previously moved to those areas because of their crime attracting qualities; or, as in many cities, because poor areas are located near commercial areas thus creating many accessible targets near home.

The attraction is created by an ecological label, often supplemented by the intending offender's personal experience and history, establishing *that* location as a known place to go for *that* kind of crime. Such crime attracting areas can also generate other types of crime that are auxiliary by-products of the intending offender having been attracted to the area by the prospect of committing the primary crime.

4.2.2.8 Road Networks; Edge Effects and Crime Corridors

The journey to crime is focused by the extant movement pathways of an area:, particularly the road network. The connectivity of the road network creates multiple paths between different places and frames the possible routes for the journey to crime (Song et al. 2019; Frith et al. 2017; Beavon et al. 1994; Weigman and Hu 1992). These tend to be dominated by collector and arterial roads which are designed to channel the flow of traffic. Arterial roads in particular are likely to become crime corridors, entering the awareness spaces of both opportunistic and information-led offenders (Wheeler et al. 2016; Wuschke et al. 2016; Beavon et al. 1994; Wilcox 1973).

Criminal events are channeled by road networks—paths of travel—into crime corridors between hot spots. Offenders travel between activity points along pathways contained in their awareness spaces, almost always moving from local roads to collector roads to arterials as their travel range increases. Along these pathways opportunistic offenders may find satisficing targets and purposive offenders may start local target searches (Brantingham and Brantingham 1981).

For any particular neighbourhood, residents and other insiders will commit crimes throughout the neighborhood while neighborhood outsiders will commit their offences near the edge, along a major pathway, but not toward the interior of the neighbourhood These have been characterized as *edge effects* (Song et al. 2015; Brantingham and Brantingham 1975) based on the permeability of neighborhoods adjacent to major pathways (Han et al. 2018; White 1990). Permeability is some function of the offender's personal awareness space; a variety of neighborhood social and economic differences from the offender's home neighborhood (Reynald et al. 2008) and the complexity of the road network through which the offender is moving (Xiao et al. 2018; Wheeler et al. 2016; Wuschke et al. 2016; Beavon et al. 1994; Weigman and Hu 1992).

4.2.3 Ecological Labels

Ecological labels—reputations popularly appended to particular places or neighborhoods—can have strong influences on where and when crimes occur An ecological label can affect who might travel to the neighborhood looking for criminal opportunities (e.g., Wright and Decker 1997). It can affect who resides in a neighborhood: attracting some, repelling others, and trapping still others. It can affect the expectations and behavior of police, housing officials, social workers and others providing services to the neighborhood, thus feeding back into the label, making the neighborhood's reputation worse (Bottoms 1994). It can affect how financial institutions deal with the neighborhood and how social researchers define issues and conduct research in the neighborhood.

It is clear that ecological labels are often at variance with actual conditions. Fear of crime in a neighborhood, for instance, may be wedded to ecological labels rather than actual crime rates (McCord et al. 2007; Rengert 1995; Nasar and Fisher 1993; Brantingham et al. 1986). Ecological labels are an important part of the backcloth against which most offenders' target selection decisions are made. Ecological labelling, however, is dynamic. Like the character of nodes, paths and edges (Brantingham and Brantingham 1993b) and like the insider/outsider distinctions useful in understanding the spatial origins of any given neighborhood's crime problem (Brantingham and Brantingham 1995a, b), the ecological label varies by level of temporal or spatial aggregation. A neighborhood could have one ecological label for daytime activity and another for night-time activity. A particular area might have a particular ecological label, but a single block within that area might have a very different label. An ecological label is a cognitive generalization. As with most cognitive processes, ecological labels can include both a limited generalization and a broader one; and both labels can exist, nested, at both levels simultaneously even as someone travels from one place to another during daily activities.

4.2.4 Hot Spot Creation

Hot spots of crime are not accidental. They are clusterings of criminal events which may seem to be independent if viewed only from the standpoint of offender decision making, but which are in fact linked to the backcloth, to general as well as specific movement and mobility patterns, and to the spatial and temporal distribution of crime generators and crime attractors. Hot spots form where different environmental criminal event predisposers, arrayed as layers of crime potentials on the environmental backcloth, overlap and intersect, building up high crime potential values. Governments unintentionally help create hot spots when they modify any of the predispositional layers for reasons wholly unrelated to crime. People make choices and take decisions that can create hot spots. Behavior is neither socially or

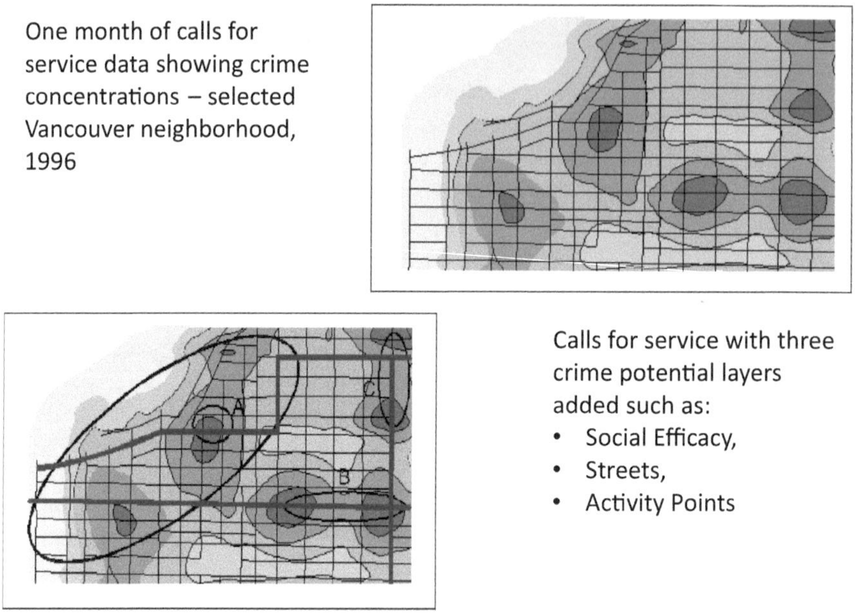

Fig. 4.6 Hot spots and crime potential layers

geographically *determined*, but human choices and decisions are made within limiting social, cultural and physical constraints. Conversely, decisions are influenced by what is easily available, by the behavior settings in which they are made and acted upon, and by fluctuations in motivation over time (Cusson 1989).

From a crime prevention perspective, understanding hot spots is useful. Figure 4.6 presents an example using some data from Vancouver, Canada. The figure does not represent an exhaustive study but is presented as a conceptual illustration of the importance of thinking about layers of crime potentials when examining crime concentrations. Figure 4.6 shows the emergence of hot spots among the set of calls for police services recorded over a one-month period in one Vancouver neighborhood in relation to different layers of crime potential.

The upper panel in Fig. 4.6 shows areas of crime concentration in a neighborhood in the northeast sector of the city. One month's worth of police calls for service data were geocoded and mapped onto a Vancouver street grid and analyzed for concentration utilizing *Mapinfo* and kernel density regionalization techniques available in the *Vertical Mapper* geostatistics package. Areas of crime concentration represented by gradations of shading from light (for low concentration) to dark (for high concentration) were plotted onto the base map to identify neighborhood hot spots. Six such hot spots are visible in the upper panel.

The second panel of Fig. 4.6 imports, integrates and plots three crime potential layers over the hot spot map. The first crime potential layer, signified by the large oval, identifies a low social efficacy residential area in this part of the city. Two of the hot spots are encompassed within this large oval.

The second crime potential layer identifies the major traffic arteries in this part of Vancouver. These roads are major routes by which commuters working in the city center traverse the neighborhood. They also act as the principal pathways for the residents of this part of the city and for workers traveling to an industrial area. Traffic is extremely light on the surrounding streets. These traffic arterials serve, then, as the primary movement paths both for neighborhood "insiders" and for "outsiders" who are just passing through. Environmental criminology would expect more crime to occur along these routes, and indeed, all six of the neighborhood hot spots are spatially associated with them.

The third crime potential layer identifies the major pedestrian activity points in the area. They are identified by small ovals labeled "A," "B," and "C" in Fig. 4.6. Oval A contains a small branch campus of a two-year post-secondary educational institution. It overlaps an arterial within the low SES area and also defines one of the neighborhood crime hot spots. Oval B is a cluster of several blocks of busy stores used by residents of this part of the city. It is arrayed along an arterial and defines two of the neighborhood's hot spots. Oval C includes a major sports arena and a large pub and defines two more neighborhood hot spots.

These layers makes it possible to see how the natural patterns of movement in the area intersect with the locations of potential offenders' residences, the location of potential targets and the location of various crime attractors and crime generators to begin the process of making a reasonable prediction of where within the neighborhood to expect concentrations of crime. This example is clearly not presented as a definitive example, but rather as an indicator of how an understanding of hotspots is tied to an understanding of the interaction of motivation, mobility, opportunity and the general backcloth.

4.2.5 A Note on Identifying Hot Spots Within Broader Crime Patterns

Crime pattern research in recent years has included a focus on development of better methods for analyzing and predicting hotspots (see, e.g., Hart, this volume; Kim and Hipp 2019; Mohler et al. 2018; Nogueira de Melo et al. 2017; Malleson and Andresen 2016; Sorg 2016; Tayebi et al. 2016; Wang et al. 2013; Johnson et al. 2008; Bowers et al. 2004).

One important approach is the use of spatial tessellation meshes, Voronoi diagrams, or Thiessen polygons centered on the micro-level locations of individual criminal events (see, e.g., Piza and Gilchrist 2018; Nogueira de Melo and Brantingham 2017; Taniguchi et al. 2011; Verma 1996). All of these techniques create polygons surrounding individual crime locations: small polygons surrounding crimes that occur in close spatial proximity and large polygons where they

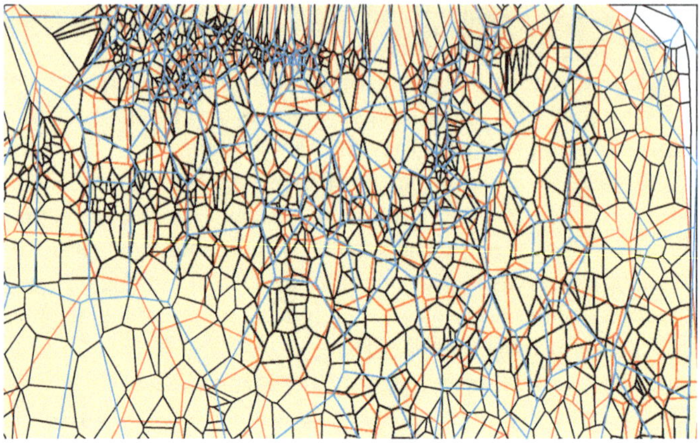

Fig. 4.7 Polygon overlays for theft, assault, and robbery

occur far apart. A crime hot spot appears as a cluster of small polygons and is quickly apparent upon inspection. Overlay of the polygons for several different offences will quickly indicate visually where multi-crime hot spots occur jointly and where hot spots for individual crime types are quite distinct (see Fig. 4.7).

Figure 4.7 illustrates this capability using address level calls for service data from a portion of Vancouver. Theft polygons are shown in black. Assault polygons are shown in blue. Robbery polygons are shown in red. As is apparent, there is a concentration for all three crime types in the upper left of the figure and a second theft corridor in the left middle of the diagram. Beyond those two concentrations, the polygons for the three crime types become progressively larger and less congruent. We believe that more extensive use of this technique by criminologists could help standardize an approach to identifying hot spots and crime corridors.

4.3 Conclusion

Hot spot analysis is important for criminology as a science and crime prevention as a policy science. Concentrations of crime in time and space are not random, but reflect individuals, their decisions, their ecological assessments of places and their actions. Crime hot spots are influenced by the environment we, as individuals, create; but they are also influenced by the environments created through lawmaking and policy setting as well as through basic land use development, transportation, marketing and social and economic conditions. Generally, crime hot spots are understandable when considered in terms of the environmental backcloth in conjunction with normal movement patterns, the distribution of crime generators and crime attractors, the situational characteristics of places and the content of ecological labels attached to different places.

Clearly more research that centers on individual criminal event behavior and how it relates to aggregate routine activities is needed if we are to refine this approach and make it into an operational crime predictor tool. Studies using spatial tessellation would be particularly helpful. Environmental criminology can be advanced with a better understanding of how people shape the environment around them, and how law, policies, government actions and the economy shape the environment in which we live. Current research seems to promise that we can develop a much better understanding of the complexity of criminal events and the complexity of crime hot spots. This research will be particularly helpful when it is associated with an expanded empirical understanding of what creates hot spots. Such improved understanding should make hot spot reduction and primary, secondary and tertiary hot spot prevention much more effective. Such understanding should eventually permit us to eradicate crime hot spots.

References

Angel, S. (1968). *Discouraging crime through city planning*. Berkeley, California: Center for Planning and Development Research, Working Paper#75.

Baldwin, J., & Bottoms, A. E. (1976). *The urban criminal*. London: Tavistock.

Barclay, P., Buckley, J., Brantingham, P. J., Brantingham, P. L., & Whin-Yates, T. (1996). Preventing auto theft in suburban Vancouver commuter lots: Effects of a bike patrol. *Crime Prevention Studies, 6*, 133–161.

Beavon, D. J. K., Brantingham, P. L., & Brantingham, P. J. (1994). The influence of street networks on the patterning of property offenses. *Crime Prevention Studies, 2*, 115–148.

Bennett, T. (1995). Identifying, explaining, and targeting burglary ‘hot spots’. *European Journal on Criminal Policy and Research, 3*, 113–123.

Bernasco, W. (2009). Foraging strategies of homo criminalis: Lessons from behavioural ecology. *Crime Patterns and Analysis, 2*, 5–16.

Bernasco, W., Ruiter, S., & Block, R. (2017). Do street robbery location choices vary over time of day or day of week? A test in Chicago. *Journal of Research in Crime and Delinquency, 54*(2), 244–275.

Block, C. R. (1990). *Hot spots and isocrimes in law enforcement decision making*. Paper presented at conference on Police and Community Responses to Drugs, University of Illinois at Chicago.

Block, C. R., & Block, R. L. (1993). *Street gang crime in Chicago*. Research in Brief, National.

Block, R. L., & Block, C. R. (1995). Space, place and crime: Hot spot areas and hot places of liquor-related crime. *Crime Prevention Studies, 4*, 145–184.

Block, R. L., & Davis, S. (1996). The environs of rapid transit stations: A focus for street crime or just another risky place? *Crime Prevention Studies, 6*, 237–257. Institute of Justice. Washington, D. C.: U.S. Department of Justice.

Boivin, R., & D’Elia, M. (2017). A network of neighborhoods: Predicting crime trips in a large canadian city. *Journal of Research in Crime and Delinquency, 54*(6), 002242781770593. https://doi.org/10.1177/0022427817705935.

Boivin, R., & Nogueira de Melo, S. (2019). The concentration of crime at place in Montreal and Toronto. *Canadian Journal of Criminology and Criminal Justice*. Advance Online Article https://doi.org/10.3138/cjccj.2018-0007.

Bottoms, A. E. (1994). Environmental criminology. In M. Maguire, R. Morgan, & R. Reiner (Eds.), *The oxford handbook of criminology*. Oxford: Clarendon Press.

Bottoms, A. E., & Wiles, P. (1986). Housing tenure and community crime careers in Britain. *Crime & Justice: A Review of Research, 8,* 101–162.
Bottoms, A. E., & Xanthos, P. (1981). Housing policy and crime in the British public sector. In P. Brantingham & P. Brantingham (Eds.), *Environmental criminology*. Beverly Hills, Calif: Sage Publications.
Bowers, K. J., Johnson, S. D., & Pease, K. (2004). Prospective hot-spotting: The future of crime mapping? *British Journal of Criminology, 44*, 641–658.
Brantingham, P. J., & Brantingham, P. L. (1984). *Patterns in crime*. New York: Macmillan Publishing Company.
Brantingham, P. L. (2006). Daily urban crime and disorder: Is there a simple solution? *Harvard International Review*. June 02, 2006.
Brantingham, P. L., & Brantingham, P. J. (1975). Residential burglary and urban form. *Urban Studies, 12,* 273–284.
Brantingham, P. L., & Brantingham, P. J. (1978). A topological technique for regionalization. *Environment and Behavior, 10,* 335–353.
Brantingham, P. L., & Brantingham, P. J. (1981). Notes on the geometry of crime. In P. Brantingham & P. Brantingham (Eds.), *Environmental criminology*. Beverly Hills, Calif: Sage Publications.
Brantingham, P. L., & Brantingham, P. J. (1993a). Environment, routine and situation: Toward a pattern theory of crime. *Advances in Criminological Theory, 5,* 259–294.
Brantingham, P. L., & Brantingham, P. J. (1993b). Nodes, paths and edges: Considerations on the complexity of crime and the physical environment *Journal of Environmental Psychology, 13*, 3–28.
Brantingham, P. L., Brantingham, P. J., & Butcher, D. (1986). Perceived and actual crime risks: An analysis of inconsistencies. In R. Figlio, S. Hakim, & G. F. Rengert (Eds.), *Metropolitan crime patterns* (pp. 139–159). Monsey, New York: Criminal Justice Press.
Brantingham, P. L., Brantingham, P. J., & Wong, P. (1990). Malls and crime: A first look. *Security Journal, 1,* 175–181.
Brantingham, P. L., Brantingham, P. J., & Wong, P. (1991). How public transit feeds private crime. *Security Journal, 2,* 91–95.
Brantingham, P. J., & Brantingham, P. L. (1995a). Environmental criminology and crime prevention. In P.-O. H. Wikstrom, R. V. Clarke, & J. McCord (Eds.), *Integrating crime prevention strategies: Propensity and opportunity*. National Council for Crime Prevention Sweden: Stockholm.
Brantingham, P. L., & Brantingham, P. J. (1995b). Criminality of place: Crime generators and crime attractors. *European Journal on Criminal Policy and Research, 3,* 5–26.
Brantingham, P. L., & Brantingham, P. J. (1999). A theoretical model of crime hot spot generation. *Studies on Crime and Crime Prevention, 8,* 7–26.
Brantingham, P. J., & Brantingham, P. L. (2013). The theory of target search. In F. Cullen & P. Wilcox (Eds.), *The oxford handbook of criminological theory* (pp. 535–553). New York: Oxford University Press.
Buckley, J. B. (1996). *Public transit and crime: A routine activities/ecological approach*. Burnaby: B.C.: Unpublished Master's thesis, Simon Fraser University.
Buerger, M. E., Cohn, E. G., & Petrosino, A. J. (1995). Defining 'hot spots of crime'; Operationalizing theoretical concepts for field research. *Crime Prevention Studies, 4,* 237–258.
Bullock, H. A. (1955). Urban homicide in theory and fact. *Journal of Criminal Law, Criminology and Police Science, 45,* 565–575.
Burgess, E. W. (1925a). The growth of the city. In R. E. Park, E. W. Burgess, & R. D. Mackenzie (Eds.), *The city*. Chicago: University of Chicago Press.
Burgess, E. W. (1925b). Can neighborhood work have a scientific basis? In R. E. Park, E. W. Burgess, & R. D. Mackenzie (Eds.), *The city*. Chicago: University of Chicago Press.
Caplan, J. M., Kennedy, L. W., & Miller, J. (2011). Risk terrain modeling: Brokering criminological theory and GIS methods for crime forecasting. *Justice Quarterly, 28*(2), 360–381.

Caplan, J. M., Kennedy, L. W., & Piza, E. L. (2013). Joint utility of event-dependent and environmental crime analysis techniques for violent crime forecasting. *Crime & Delinquency, 59*(2), 243–270.

Capone, D., & Nichols, W. (1976). Urban structure and criminal mobility. *American Behavioral Scientist, 20,* 199–201.

Coburn, G. (1988). *Patterns of homicide in Vancouver*, 1980–1986. Unpublished M.A. Thesis, Simon Fraser University. Burnaby, British Columbia: Simon Fraser University.

Cornish, D. (1994). The procedural analysis of offending and its relevance for situational prevention. *Crime Prevention Studies, 3*, 151–196.

Costanzo, C. M., Halperin, W. C., & Gale, N. (1986). Criminal mobility and the directional component in journeys to crime. In Figlio, R. M., Hakim, S., & Rengert, G. F. (Eds.), *Metropolitan crime patterns*. Monsey, New York: Criminal Justice Press.

Cromwell, P. F., Olson, J. N., & Avary, D. W. (1991). *Breaking and entering: An ethnographic analysis of burglary*. Newbury Park, Ca.: Sage Publications.

Curman, A. S. N., Andresen, M. A., & Brantingham, P. J. (2015). Crime and place: A longitudinal examination of street segment patterns in Vancouver, BC. *Journal of Quantitative Criminology, 31*, 127–147.

Cusson, M. (1989). Les zones urbaines criminelles. *Criminologie, 22,* 95–105.

Demeau, E., & Parent, G. (2018). Impacts of crime attractors and generators on criminality in Montreal. *Canadian Journal of Criminology and Criminal Justice., 60*(3), 1–26.

Deryol, R., Wilcox, P., Logan, M., & Wooldredge, J. (2016). Crime places in context: An illustration of the multilevel nature of hot spot development. *Journal of Quantitative Criminology, 32,* 305–325.

Eck, J. E. (1996). Preventing crime at places. In L. W. Sherman, D. Gottfredson, D. MacKenzie, J. Eck, P. Reuter, & S. Bushway (Eds.), *Preventing crime: What works, what doesn't, what's promising: A report to the United States congress*. Web document found at http://www.ncjrs.org/works/chapter7.htm.

Edmunds, M., Hough, M., & Urquía, N. (1996). *Tackling local drug markets*. Crime Detection and Prevention Series, Paper 80. London: Home Office Police Research Group.

Engstad, P. A. (1975). Environmental opportunities and the ecology of crime. In R. A. Silverman & J. J. Teevan Jr. (Eds.), *Crime in Canadian society*. Toronto: Butterworths.

Feeney, F. (1986). Robbers as decision makers. In D. Cornish, & R. Clarke (Eds.), *The reasoning criminal* (pp. 53–71). New York: Springer.

Felson, M. (1994). *Crime and everyday life: Insight and implications for society*. Thousand Oaks, CA: Pine Forge Press.

Fink, G. (1969). Einsbruchstatorte vornehmlich an einfallstrassen? *Kriminalistik, 23,* 358–360.

Fleming, Z., Brantingham, P. L., Brantingham, P. J. (1994). Exploring auto theft in British Columbia. *Crime Prevention Studies, 3*, 47–91.

Frank, R., Dabbaghian, V., Singh, S., Reid, A., Cinnamon, J., & Brantingham, P. (2011). Power of criminal attractors: Modeling the pull of activity nodes. *Journal of Artificial Societies and Social Simulation, 14*(1), 6. Access at http://jasss.soc.surrey.ac.uk/14/1/6.

Frith, M. J., Johnson, S. D., & Fry, H. M. (2017). Role of the street network in Burglars spatial decision making. *Criminology, 55*(2), 344–376.

Gabor, T., Baril, M., Cusson, M., Elie, D., LeBlanc, M., & Normandeau, A. (1987). *Armed robbery: Cops, robbers and victims*. Springfield, Illinois: Charles C. Thomas.

Haberman, C. P. (2017). Overlapping hot spots? Examination of the spatial heterogeneity of hot spots of different crime types. *Criminology & Public Policy, 16*(2), 633–660.

Hakim, S., Rengert, G., & Shachmurove, Y. (2001). Target search of burglars: A revised economic model. *Papers in Regional Science, 80,* 121–137.

Han, Y., Zhua, X., Ye, X., Hub, T., & Kudvad, S. (2018). Modelling the effects of street permeability on burglary in Wuhan, China. *Applied Geography, 98,* 177–183.

Hesseling, R. (1995). Theft from cars: Reduced or displaced?. *European Journal on Criminal Policy and Research, 3,* 79–92.

Hipp, J. R., & Young-An, K. (2019). Explaining the temporal and spatial dimensions of robbery: Differences across measures of the physical and social environment. *Journal of Criminal Justice, 60*(1), 1–12.

Hirschfield, A., Bowers, K. J., & Brown, P. J. B. (1995). Exploring relations between crime and disadvantage on Merseyside. *European Journal on Criminal Policy and Research, 3,* 93–112.

Jacobs, B. A. (2010). Serendipity in robbery target selection. *The British Journal of Criminology, 50,* 514–529.

Johnson, S. D., Lab, S. P., & Bowers, K. J. (2008). Stable and fluid hotspots of crime: Differentiation and identification. *Built Environment, 34*(1), 32–45.

Johnson, S. D., Summers, L., Pease, K. (2009). Offender as forager? A direct test of the boost account of victimization. *Journal of Quantitative Criminology, 25,* 181–200.

Kim, Y.-A., & Hipp, J. R. (2019). Street Egohood: An alternative perspective of measuring neighborhood and spatial patterns of crime. *Journal of Quantitative Criminology.*

Kinney, J. B., Brantingham, P. L., Wuschke, K., Kirk, Michael G., & Brantingham, Paul J. (2008). Crime attractors, generators and detractors: Land use and urban crime opportunities. *Built Environment, 34*(1), 62–74.

Langworthy, R. H., & Le Beau, J. (1992a). The spatial evolution of a sting clientele. *Journal of Criminal Justice, 20,* 135–146.

Langworthy, R. H., & Le Beau, J. (1992b). The spatial distribution of sting targets. *Journal of Criminal Justice, 20,* 541–552.

LeBeau, J. L. (1995). The temporal ecology of calls for police service. In C. R. Block, M. Dabdoub, & S. Fregly (Eds.), *Crime analysis through computer mapping*. Washington, D.C.: Police Executive Research Forum.

Lee, Y. J., Eck, J. E., Soo Hyun, O., & Martinez, N. N. (2017). How concentrated is crime at places? A systematic review from 1970 to 2015. *Crime Science, 6,* 6. https://doi.org/10.1186/s40163-017-0069-x.

Lowe, J. C., & Moryadas, S. (1975). *The geography of movement*. Boston: Houghton Mifflin.

Maguire, M. (1982). *Burglary in a dwelling*. London: Heinemann.

Malleson, N., & Andresen, M. A. (2016). Exploring the impact of ambient population measures on London crime hotspots. *Journal of Criminal Justice, 46,* 52–63.

McCord, E. S., Ratcliffe, J. H., Garcia, R. M., & Taylor, R. B. (2007). Nonresidential crime attractors and generators elevate perceived neighborhood crime and incivilities. *Journal of Research in Crime and Delinquency, 44*(3), 295–320.

Menting, B. (2018). Awareness × opportunity: Testing interactions between activity nodes and criminal opportunity in predicting crime location choice. *British Journal of Criminology, 58*(5), 1171–1192.

Mohler, G., Brantingham, P. J., Carter, J., & Short, M. (2018). *Unbiased estimation of the law of crime concentration*. Preprint.

Morris, T. (1958). *The criminal area: A study in social ecology*. London: Routledge and Kegan Paul.

Nasar, J. L., & Fisher, B. (1993). Hot spots of fear and crime: A multi-method investigation. *Journal of Environmental Psychology, 13,* 187–206.

Nogueira de Melo, S., Frank, R., & Brantingham, P. L. (2017). Voronoi diagrams and spatial analysis of crime. *The Professional Geographer, 69*(4), 579–590.

Perry, S. (2019). The application of the "Law of Crime Concentration" to terrorism: The Jerusalem case study. *Journal of Quantitative Criminology.* https://doi.org/10.1007/s10940-019-09411-2.

Piza, E. L., & Gilchrist, A. M. (2018). Measuring the effect heterogeneity of police enforcement actions across spatial contexts. *Journal of Criminal Justice, 54,* 76–87.

Pyle, G. F. (1974). *The spatial dynamics of crime*. Chicago: Department of Geography, University of Chicago.

Reid, A., Frank, R., Iwanski, N., Dabbaghian, V., & Brantingham, P. L. (2014). Uncovering the spatial patterning of crimes: A criminal movement model (CriMM). *Journal of Research in Crime and Delinquency, 51,* 230–255.

Rengert, G. F. (1994). Drogue et crime: L'impact du commerce de drogues sur le tissu urbain. *Criminologie, 27,* 69–79.
Rengert, G. F. (1995). Comparing cognitive hot spots to crime hot spots. In C. R. Block, M. Dabdoub, & S. Fregly (Eds.), *Crime analysis through computer mapping*. Washington, D.C.: Police Executive Research Forum.
Rengert, G. F., & Wasilchick, T. (1985). *Suburban Burglary*. Springfield, Illinois: Charles C. Thomas.
Reynald, D., Averdijk, M., Elffers, H., & Bernasco, W. (2008). Do social barriers affect urban crime trips? The effects of ethnic and economic neighborhood compositions on the flow of crime in The Hague, The Netherlands. *Built Environment, 34*(1), 21–31.
Rhodes, W. M., & Conly, C. (1991). Crime and mobility: An empirical study. In P. Brantingham & P. Brantingham (Eds.), *Environmental criminology*. Prospect Heights, Illinois: Waveland Press.
Roncek, D., & Maier, P. A. (1991). Bars, blocks and crime revisited: Linking the theory of routine activities to the empiricism of hot spots. *Criminology, 29,* 725–753.
Rossmo, D. K. (1994). Targeting victims: Serial killers and the urban environment. In T. O'Reilly-Fleming & S. Egger (Eds.), *Serial and mass murder: Theory, research and policy*. Toronto: University of Toronto Press.
Schmid, C. (1960a). Urban crime areas - Part I. *American Sociological Review, 25*, 527–543.
Schmid, C. (1960b). Urban crime areas - Part II. *American Sociological Review, 25*, 655–678.
Shaw, C. R. (1929). *Delinquency areas*. Chicago: University of Chicago Press.
Shaw, C., & McKay, H. D. (1942). *Delinquency and urban areas*. Chicago: University of Chicago Press.
Sherman, L. W., Gartin, P. R., & Buerger, M. E. (1989). Hot spots of predatory crime: Routine activities and the criminology of place. *Criminology, 27*, 27–55.
Sherman, L. W., & Weisburd, D. (1995). General deterrent effects of police patrol in crime 'hot spots': A randomized, controlled trial. *Justice Quarterly, 12*, 625.
Song, G., Bernasco, W., Liu, L., Xiao, L., Zhou, S., & Liao, W. (2019). Crime feeds on legal activities: Daily mobility flows help to explain thieves' target location choices. *Journal of Quantitative Criminology*. https://doi.org/10.1007/s10940-019-09406-z—published online February 13, 2019.
Song, J., Andresen, M., Brantingham, P. L., & Spicer, V. (2015). Crime on the edges: Patterns of crime and land use change. *Cartography and Geographic Information Science, 44*(1), 51–61.
Sorg, E. T. (2016). Classifying import and domestic hot spots of crime by offender home proximity. *Policing, 10*(3), 264–277.
Spicer, V., Song, J., Brantingham, P. L., & Andresen, M. (2016). Street profile analysis: A new method for mapping crime on major roadways. *Applied Geography, 69,* 65–74.
Taniguchi, T. A., Ratcliffe, J. H., & Taylor, R. B. (2011). Gang set space, drug markets, and crime around drug corners in Camden. *Journal of Research in Crime & Delinquency*, *48*(3), 327–363.
Tayebi, M., Glässer, U., Ester, M., & Brantingham, P. L. (2016). Personalized crime location prediction. *European Journal of Applied Mathematics, 27*(03), 422–450.
Verma, A. (1996). *New tools of analysis in quantitative criminology: An exploration. Burnaby, British Columbia*: Unpublished Ph. D. Dissertation, Simon Fraser University.
Verma, A., Mu, S., Brantingham, P. L., & Brantingham, P. J. (1994). *The ecological rhythms and routines of crime in Vancouver*. Paper read at American Society of Criminology, Miami.
Wang, D., Ding, W., Lo, H., Stepinski, T., Salazar, J., & Morabito, M. (2013) Crime hotspot mapping using the crime related factors—A spatial data mining approach. *Applied Intelligence, 39*, 772–781.
Weigman, F., & Hu, D. (1992). *An analysis of auto theft in Vancouver using the network capabilities of the arc info geographic information system*. Burnaby: British Columbia Institute of Technology.
Weisburd, D. (2015). The law of crime concentration and crime and justice practice. *Criminology, 53*(2), 133–157.

Weisburd, D., Green, L., & Ross, D. (1994). Analyse spatiale des crimes comis sur la rue à l'intérier des marchés de drogues. *Criminologie, 27,* 49–67.

Weisburd, D. L., Groff, E. R., & Yang, S. M. (2012). *The criminology of place: Street segments and our understanding of the crime problem.* New York: Oxford University Press.

Weisburd, D., Maher, L., Sherman, L., Buerger, M., Cohn, E., & Petrosino, A. (1993). Contrasting crime general and crime specific theory: The case of hot spots of crime. *Advances in Criminological Theory, 4,* 45–70.

Wheeler, A. P., Worden, R. E., & McLean, S. J. (2016). Replicating group-based trajectory models of crime at micro-places in Albany, NY. *Journal of Quantitative Criminology, 32,* 589–612.

White, G. F. (1990). Neighborhood permeability and burglary rates. *Justice Quarterly, 7,* 57–67.

Wikstrom, P.-O. H. (1985). *Everyday violence in contemporary Sweden: Situational and ecological aspects.* Stockholm: The National Council for Crime Prevention Sweden.

Wikstrom, P.-O. H. (1991). *Urban crime, criminals and victims: The Swedish experience in an anglo-american comparative perspective.* New York: Springer.

Wilcox, S. (1973). *The geography of robbery.* [The Prevention and Control of Robbery, Vol. 3]. Davis: The Center of Administration of Justice, University of California at Davis.

Wright, R. T., & Decker, S. H. (1997). *Armed robbers in action: Stickups and street culture.* Boston: Northeastern University Press.

Wuschke, K., Song, J., & Spicer, V. (2016). Crime in the built urban environment: Exploring the impact of road networks and land use on residential burglary patterns. Posted at *summit.sfu.ca.*

Xiao, L., Liu, L., Song, G., Ruiter, S., & Zhou, S. (2018). Journey-to-crime distances of residential burglars in China disentangled: Origin and destination effects. *ISPRS International Journal of Geo-Inf*ormation, *7,* 325–349.

Chapter 5
Hot Spots of Crime: Methods and Predictive Analytics

Timothy C. Hart

As part of a contemporary look at the intersection of geography and crime, the current chapter offers a new conceptual definition of predictive policing, an overview of some of the most commonly used methods to identify crime "hot spots" retrospectively, prospective hot spot analysis, and predictive policing analytics. Police and researchers have mapped crime and disorder for decades, consistently finding that these incidents clusters in areas commonly referred to as hot spots. Understanding where and when crime and disorder cluster, both spatially and temporally, provides vital information necessary for community leaders to design and implement effective crime-reduction strategies and community-safety initiatives. Until recently, however, researchers and analysts have operated *retrospectively*—using incident location information to describe historical crime patterns through the use of data visualization techniques or to design reactionary policing strategies based on the assumption that historical crime patterns are reliable indicators of future problem areas. Unlike traditional crime hot spot analysis, predictive analytics identify patterns in crime data that relate to criminal activity in the near future. The aim of this approach is to exploit patterns identified in data dynamically and to prevent crime through *proactive* resource allocation. This approach is distinct from how crime analysis and intelligence-led policing has historically been conducted.

T. C. Hart (✉)
University of Tampa, 401 W. Kennedy Blvd., Science Wing, Plant Hall 255, Tampa, FL 33606, USA
e-mail: thart@ut.edu

K. M. Lersch and J. Chakraborty (eds.), *Geographies of Behavioural Health, Crime, and Disorder*, GeoJournal Library 126,
https://doi.org/10.1007/978-3-030-33467-3_5

5.1 Defining Predictive Policing

Intelligence-led policing has grown as more agencies integrate geographic information systems (GIS) into their crime-fighting efforts. As agencies become more sophisticated and move beyond retrospective hot spot analyses, several techniques for predicting the time and location of crimes are becoming more commonplace. Although a growing number of agencies use GIS to advance their crime-fighting efforts through predictive policing, there is no universally accepted definition of predictive policing. Nevertheless, several definitions have been proposed and each stress the important role that data analytics plays in the modern predictive policing process. For example, the Rand Corporation defines predictive policing as…

> The application of analytic techniques–particularly quantitative techniques–to identify likely targets for police intervention and prevent crime or solve past crimes by making statistical predictions (Perry et al. 2013, pp. 1–2).

Extant definitions of predictive policing also describe it as a data-driven management strategy, based on prospective forecasts, which aims to detect and reduce crime through police resource allocation:

> The use of historical data to create a spatiotemporal forecast of areas of criminality or crime hot spots that will be the basis for police resource allocation decisions with the expectation that having officers at the proposed place and time will deter or detect criminal activity (Ratcliffe 2014, p. 4).

More recent definitions of predictive policing highlight how predictive policing can be viewed as part of a broader approach to crime fighting that leverages administrative data, applying advanced analytic techniques, and involving targeted intervention strategies. For example, Brantingham (2018) defines predictive policing as a three-part process where…

> (1) data of one or more type are ingested; (2) algorithmic methods use ingested data to forecast the occurrence of crime in some domain of interest; and (3) police use forecasts to inform strategic and tactical decisions in the field (p. 473).

Considering these and other definitions, Birks et al. (2019) recently offered the following description of predictive policing:

> The use of dynamic prediction models that apply spatiotemporal algorithms to administrative data with the purpose of forecasting areas and times of increased crime risk, which could be targeted by law enforcement agencies with associated prevention strategies designed to mitigate and/or reduce those risks.

The definition offered by Birks and colleagues is distinguishable from traditional crime hot spot mapping techniques because it emphasizes the importance of three fundamental components of predictive policing: (1) dynamic prediction models that rely on advanced algorithms; (2) near term forecasts of elevated crime risk; and (3) the use of this information to inform crime reduction strategies.

Predicting the locations and times of future crime events is of great interest to law enforcement agencies and academics around the world. Although predictive policing is a relatively new way to analyze crime data, several methods and techniques designed to forecast crime patterns exist. These include crime hot spot mapping, regression methods, near-repeat analysis, spatiotemporal analysis, cluster analysis, and risk terrain modelling. Regardless of method used to forecast crime, the ultimate goal of predictive policing is to inform a proactive approach to crime prevention. Traditional hot spot methods and the ways in which they differ from modern predictive policing techniques, including those applied in the current study, are described in the next section.

5.2 Retrospective Hot Spot Analysis

A growing number of analysts and academics from around the world study crime data patterns to identify crime hot spots and to convey these patterns visually, in the form of hot spot maps. Crime hot spots are areas of concentrated incident locations that demonstrate a nonrandom pattern in space or time. Depending on the size of the geographic area being studied (e.g., address locations, streets, blocks, suburbs, jurisdictions, etc.) and the particular research question at hand, different types of hot spot methods can be employed. A variety of techniques has emerged from the academic literature over the past several years (Bowers et al. 2004; Chainey and Ratcliffe 2005; Eck et al. 2005) and can be grouped into two generally categories: methods based on aggregated incident locations and analysis of point-patterns.

5.2.1 Local Tests of Spatial Association

Crime hot spot techniques that rely on aggregated crime counts include grid-based thematic mapping and local tests of spatial association. Two of the most common tests of spatial association used in crime analysis are Local Moran's I (Anselin 1995) and Gi*/Getis-Ord local statistic (Getis and Ord 1992; Ord and Getis 1995). Although both of these aggregate tests of statistical association are unique, they generally follow a similar approach. Correlation statistics are calculated for each areal unit based on aggregated crime counts and the statistics are weighted by a spatial matrix that is defined by the locations and distances of neighboring crime counts. For example, Eqs. (5.1–5.5) are used to calculate the Local Moran's I statistic (Anselin 1995) of spatial association and is given as:

$$I_i = \frac{x_i - \bar{X}}{S_i^2} \sum_{j=1, j \neq i}^{n} w_{i,j}(x_i - \bar{X}) \tag{5.1}$$

where x_i is an attribute for feature I, $\bar{X}$ is the mean of the corresponding attribute, $w_{i,j}$ is the spatial weight between feature i and j, and:

$$s_i^2 = \frac{\sum_{j=1, j \neq i}^{n} w_{ij}}{n - 1} = \bar{X}^2 \tag{5.2}$$

with n equating to the total number of features.

The z_{I_i}-score for the statistics are computed as follows:

$$z_{I_i} = \frac{I_i - \mathrm{E}[I_i]}{\sqrt{\mathrm{V}[I_i]}} \tag{5.3}$$

where:

$$\mathrm{E}[I_i] = \frac{\sum_{j=1, j \neq i}^{n}}{n - 1} \tag{5.4}$$

$$V[I_i] = \mathrm{E}\left[I_i^2\right] - \mathrm{E}[I_i]^2 \tag{5.5}$$

Aggregate tests of statistical association like this are used to identify patterns in crime incident data based on historical information and to determine whether clusters of incidents are arranged in significant, nonrandom patterns across a study area. With Anselin's Local Moran's I, for example, crime patterns are defined by classifying output into one of five distinct groups: a High-High (HH) group, defined by high crime counts clustering around other neighboring high crime counts and that are above the average value; a Low-Low (LL) group, defined by low values clustering around other low values and that are below the average; a High-Low (HL) group, where high values cluster with low values and that are below the mean; a Low-High (LH) group, where low values cluster around high values and that are below the mean; and finally, an insignificant group, where no significant clustering is observed (Anselin 1995). When interpreting these results, the first two groups (i.e., the HH and LL group) represent positive spatial autocorrelation. Conversely, the 3rd and 4th group (i.e., the HL and LH group) reflect negative spatial autocorrelation. These two groups are also referred as outliers or dissimilar values.

5.2.2 *Point Pattern Analysis*

An alternative approach to crime hot spot mapping involves point-pattern analysis. These techniques are also referred to as adaptive scanning methods. Point-pattern methods include modal hot spot analysis, nearest neighbor hierarchical clustering (NNH) (Hartigan 1975; Ward 1963), spatial and temporal analysis of crime (STAC) (Spring and Block 1989), and K-means clustering (Ball and Hall 1970; McBratney and deBruijter 1992; Thompson 1956). Like aggregate methods for determining spatial associations, points-pattern techniques share a common approach: identifying spatially clustered discrete crime event locations, based on certain input parameters used to conceptualize a crime hot spot.

For example, NNH methods, which are among the oldest hierarchical clustering techniques used in point-pattern analysis (Johnson 1967; D'Andrade 1978) require several criteria to be defined before the data can be analyzed. These criteria include the threshold distance, the minimum number of points that define a "cluster", and how results will be visually displayed. As the name suggests, the threshold distance criterion is used to define how close data points are required to be in order to form a cluster. This information is used in conjunction with the second criterion, the minimum number of point that define a cluster, to construct groups of clustered data points. Finally, results of NNH analysis visually display crime hot spots as geometrically defined areas such as ellipses and convex hulls.

Similarly, STAC parameter settings include the size of the search radius, the units in which the search radius is based, the minimum number of points that define a cluster, the number of simulations that will be run (if Monet Carlo simulations are utilized), the type of scanning procedure (e.g., rectangular or triangular), and the number of standard deviations used to create the output ellipses (Bates 1987; Canter 1993; Spring and Block 1989). Like NNH and aggregated incident location methods, results of point patterns, including those produced from STAC, are based solely on historical crime data and therefore offer limited insight into where crime may occur in the future because they are entirely retrospective in nature.

5.3 Prospective Hot Spot Methods

Many traditional crime hot spot techniques use crime incident location information to describe retrospective crime patterns. However, other methods use historical data to produce prospective hot spot maps, based on the assumption that past crime hot spots are reliable indicators of future problem areas. For example, using repeat/near-repeat analysis on burglary data collected in Brisbane, Australia, Townsley et al. (2003) demonstrated how the chance of a residential burglary can more than double after an initial burglary and that this elevated risk extends to nearby locations. However, their findings provided greater support for the near repeat hypothesis among suburban homes that were defined by dwellings that were more dissimilar in appearance than among homes that were more homogeneous. These types of short-term forecasts of crime risk permit the implementation of policing strategies to proactively address problem areas or times. Furthermore, findings such as these have been consistently observed across different crime types (e.g., robbery, burglary, aggravated assaults, and auto theft) and in several different countries (e.g., Australia, U.S., and Europe).

5.3.1 Repeat (R) and Near Repeat (NR) Analysis

Repeat (R) and near repeat (NR) patterns can be identified in crime data and used to address problem areas and times, proactively. R/NR patterns are defined as the likelihood of people or targets to be victimized more than once being greater than the likelihood of someone or someplace being victimized for the first time (Groff and Taniguchi 2018; Townsley et al. 2003). Two explanations have been offered to better understand R/NR patterns.

First, the boost account suggests that R/NR crime patterns emerge in data as a result of the same offender returning to where he or she succeeded at committing his or her initial offense. The boost account explanation is based on optimal foraging theory (Fielding and Jones 2012; Johnson and Bowers 2004), which is based on a simple risk-reward assessment of the situation: time and effort (and risk of apprehension) should be diminished, while benefit and reward should be maximized (Johnson et al. 2009). An alternative explanation of R/NR is the flag account (Tseloni and Pease 2003). The flag account suggests it is the characteristics of the person/target that entice potential offenders, but that these characteristics remain constant over time. Simply put, the boot account explains repeat patterns in crime data in terms of the offender, whereas the flag account explains it in terms of the target or victim.

The most common approach to identifying R/NR patterns is through the application of the Near Repeat Calculator (Ratcliffe 2007), shown in Fig. 5.1. The Near Repeat Calculator is available online through Temple University's Center for Security and Crime Science and can be distributed for educational purposes at no cost. To analyze suspected patterns in crime data using the Near Repeat Calculator, a user simply provides a crime data file in .csv format that contains three characteristics for each incident: (1) the latitude coordinate; (2) the longitude coordinate; and (3) the date of the incident. After the crime data file is opened in the calculator, the user sets four parameters that guide the R/NR analysis: (1) the spatial bandwidth; (2) the number of spatial bands; (3) the temporal bandwidth; and (4) the

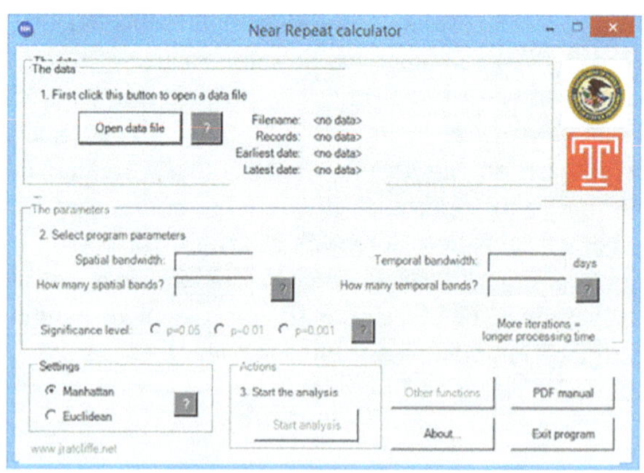

Fig. 5.1 Ratcliffe's (2007) near repeat calculator interface

number of temporal bands. The researcher or crime analyst can also set the significant level, choosing between a null-hypothesis rejection threshold of $p = 0.05$; $p = 0.10$; and $p = 0.01$ (Ratcliffe 2007; Ratcliffe and Rengert 2008).

The first two parameters, the spatial bandwidth and the number of spatial bands, are used to determine whether spatial patterns exist in the data. In order to make observed spatial patterns in the data easier to interpret, they are disaggregated into distance bands (i.e., spatial bands) (Ratcliffe 2007). For example, if each block in a study area is about 400 ft, then a spatial bandwidth of 400 ft might be appropriate. This will allow the user to understand the output in terms a certain number of blocks, which would be reflection a feature (i.e., city blocks) found in the urban landscape.

The number of spatial bands is used to quantify how far R/NR patterns in the data are expected to extend across the landscape (Ratcliffe 2007). If, for example, R/NR patterns are believed to extend 1600 ft and a distance band is set at 400 ft, then the number of spatial bands would be set at four (i.e., 4 bands × 400 ft bandwidth = 1600 ft distance). In short, the spatial distance, divided by the spatial bandwidth, produces the number of spatial bands that will be used by the Near Repeat Calculator in its analysis of the crime data that the researcher or analyst inputs.

The temporal bands and bandwidths use a similar logic, but are applied to identify temporal patterns in the data (Ratcliffe 2007). The temporal bandwidth refers to the length of time after the initial crime occurs that the program will "search" for repeat incidents. This parameter can be set at number of days (i.e., 7 days, 14 days, 21 days, etc.). Bandwidths commonly used in previous research included one week, two weeks, and one month. Finally, users must determine the how long to continue to search for patterns (i.e., how many days) and divide this temporal distance by the number of temporal bandwidths to establish the number of temporal bands to use in the analysis. This is comparable to how the number of spatial bands is determined (e.g., 13 bands × 14-day bandwidth = 6-month time period) (Short et al. 2009).

When output from the Near Repeat Calculator is produced, distances are reported as either straight-line distance (i.e., Euclidean distance) or grid-based distance (i.e., Manhattan distance). Grid-based distances are typically used when the analyst or researcher wants to represent street networks. Regardless of how distances are reported, the calculator presents them in a simple R/NR table, where table columns denote time (i.e., temporal bandwidths) and the table rows reflect distances (i.e., spatial bandwidths). Each table cell indicates the likelihood of another victimization occurring at that time/distance, following an initial incident, based on the crime data provided; times and distances that are significantly higher than expected likelihoods of repeat victimization (or near repeat victimizations) are color coded for easy identification (Ratcliffe 2007).

5.3.2 Kernel Density Estimation (KDE)

Kernel Density Estimation (KDE) is another popular alternative to retrospective crime mapping techniques. With KDE, a prospective risk map is created with *interpolated* data derived from known crime incident location information and their associated spatial coordinates. The KDE process generalizes or "smooths" these discrete data points so that a continuous surface area is produced and visualized (Bailey and Gatrell 1995). Put simply, KDE involves estimating the density of crime across an entire two-dimensional study area, based on the known locations of discrete events.

KDE begins by overlaying a grid (with *n* equally sized cells) on top of the study area and calculating a density estimate based on the center points of each grid cell. Each distance between an incident and the center of a grid cell is then weighted based on a specific method of interpolation (i.e., the kernel function) and bandwidth (i.e., search radius). Figure 5.2 illustrates the KDE process and shows a number of parameters that must be considered before a density estimate can be produced. These parameters include the grid cell size, the method of interpolation, and the bandwidth.[1]

As previously mentioned, KDE begins the interpolation process by overlaying a two-dimensional grid (with *n* equally sized cells) across an entire study area. One of the first parameters that must be established, therefore, is how large to make each cell. Decision rules about grid-cell size or the number of columns into which the grid overlay will be divided[2] are usually based the size of the study area. In general, KDE maps with greater resolution (i.e., less pixilation) are produced from grid overlays with smaller cells (i.e., more columns), whereas maps with less resolution result when grid overlays are comprised of larger sized cells (i.e., fewer columns). Variations in one or more of these parameter settings have been shown to drastically affect KDE output (Hart and Zandbergen 2012, 2014), as illustrated in Fig. 5.3.

Although debate over whether KDE consistently outperforms other prospective hotspot techniques is ongoing (see, for example, Levine 2008; Pezzuchi 2008; Chainey et al. 2008a, b, c), past research suggests that KDE can be used to accurately and reliably describe areas most vulnerable to crime. As a result, it has

[1]In KDE, bandwidths are defined as either "adaptive" or "fixed interval." Adaptive bandwidths are typically used when a sample of point locations are used in lieu of all points located within the study area, which is generally not the case in crime analysis. If adaptive bandwidths are used, the minimum sample size is an additional parameter that must be defined. Fixed interval bandwidths, on the other hand, are used when the entire population of events is analyzed (e.g., all crimes within a given timeframe). When a fixed interval bandwidth is selected, the size of the bandwidth must be defined (Brunsdon 1995).

[2]Instead of asking users to define the actual cell size, most GIS applications that include KDE as an analytic method for identifying hot spots (e.g., ArcGIS and MapInfo) ask the user to indicate how many columns the grid overlay should be divided into. This input value is then used to calculate the actual size of each grid cell.

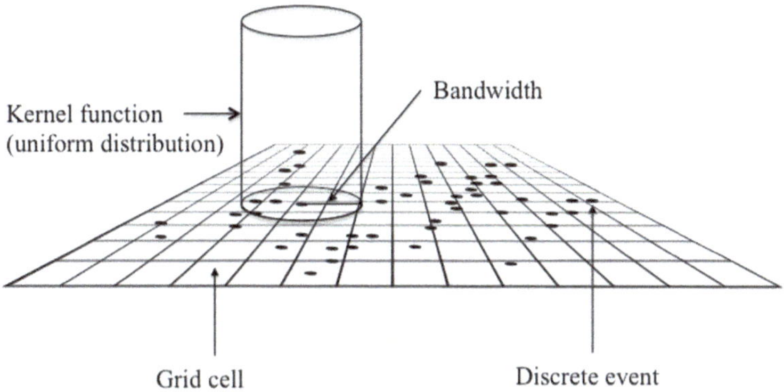

Fig. 5.2 The KDE process uses discrete data points to interpolate a continuous risk surface, based on a number of parameters that must be defined by the analyst or researcher

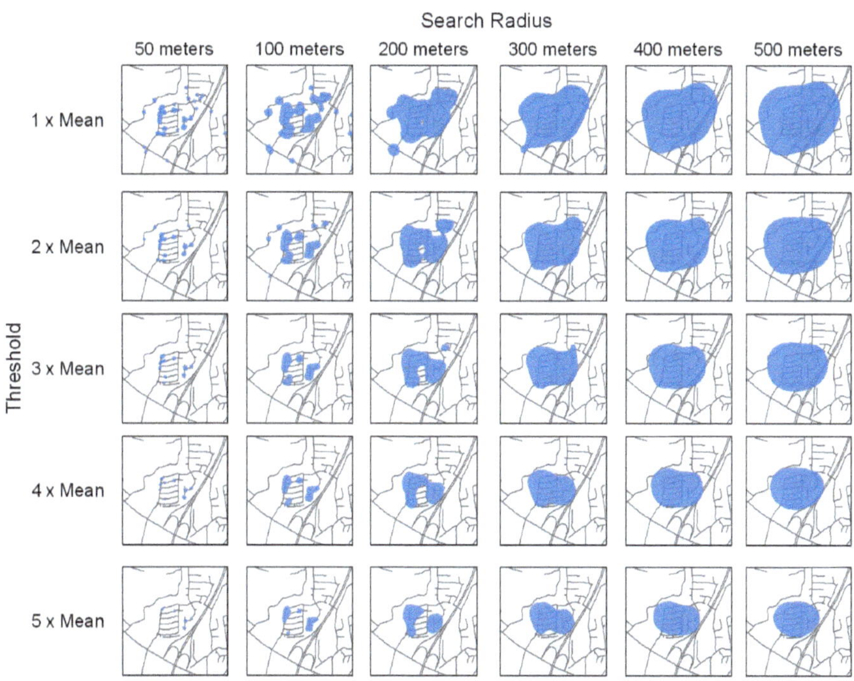

Fig. 5.3 Hart and Zandbergen (2012) show how changes in two KDE parameters (i.e., the search radius and threshold setting) can impact how KDE results are visually depicted

become a popular approach to visualize crime hot spots. Tools used to create KDE maps are available in all of the major software packages used in crime analysis, including leading commercial GIS products (e.g., ArcGIS and MapInfo) and other non-commercial spatial statistics applications (e.g., R and CrimeStatIV [Levine

2015]). Perhaps one of the most popular applications of KDE to produce prospective crime hot spot maps is Risk Terrain Modeling (RTM) (Caplan and Kennedy 2010; Caplan et al. 2011).

5.3.3 *Risk Terrain Modeling (RTM)*

Risk Terrain Modeling (RTM) identifies the spatial influence of multiple risk factors within a specific geographic area, including crime incident locations, to inform decisions about factors that are used to model an area's risk of crime. These risk factors are used to create separate KDE map layers that are combined to produce a composite risk terrain map (Caplan and Kennedy 2010; Caplan and Kennedy 2010). A large and growing body empirical research demonstrates how theoretically- and empirically-grounded risk terrain maps can articulate micro-level places where conditions are suitable for crime, given the existing environmental context (e.g., Barnum et al. 2017; Caplan and Kennedy 2010; Caplan and Kennedy 2010, 2013; Drawve and Barnum 2015; Edmonds and Mallard 2011; Garnier et al. 2018; Yerxa 2013). One of the most recent applications of this innovative approach involved a multi-city risk-based policing project where RTM was used to address myriad crime-related problems (Piza et al. 2018).

To date, RTM software has been used in over 45 countries and in more than two-thirds of all of the United States. One features of RTM that makes it especially appealing to law enforcement agencies is the Risk Terrain Modeling Diagnostics Utility (RTMDx), a self-contained program developed through funding from the National Institute of Justice (NIJ) and available through Rutgers University's Center on Public Security. The RTMDx program makes it relatively easy to identify areas of elevated risk for criminal activity because it requires the user to input just a few data files that are relatively easy to obtain (Fig. 5.4)..

To produce a risk terrain map, a user must first obtain a polygon "shapefile" that corresponds to a study area's boundary. RTM can be used to analyze risk across a variety of landscapes, so different polygon shapefiles can be used, including those that represent census tracts, patrol beats, agency jurisdictions, or an entire municipality. The projected shapefile that define the study area will serve as the reference layer for orienting and analyzing the other data files used in the RTM analysis. Fortunately, local governments, especially those that serve large populations, often provide shapefiles online at no cost. Shapefiles that define official administrative boundaries (e.g., census tracts) are also available online through the U.S. Census Bureau's website. Finally, law enforcement agencies that oversee large jurisdictions often provide polygon shapefiles online for free and that contain information corresponding to patrol boundaries, which can be used to better contextualize RTM results from a law enforcement perspective.

Data that correspond to the topic being studies are also needed to run the RTMDx utility. The topic data will correspond to a problem(s) or issue(s) that is the focus of one's investigation (e.g., incident locations of robberies, traffic crashes, or

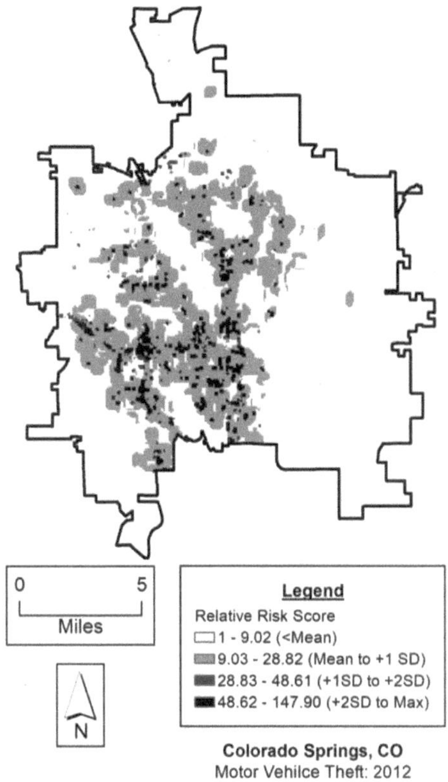

Fig. 5.4 RTM map showing areas of elevated risk of motor vehicle thefts in Colorado Springs, CO (Piza et al. 2018)

drug overdoses). These data must be spatially referenced or have location information that will allow them to be accurately geocoded (Hart and Zandbergen 2012, 2013). It is also recommended that topic data is representative of the entire study area.

Finally, risk-factor data is needed to run the RTMDx utility. According to the Caplan et al. (2011), these data represent environmental features found in the study area that may represent crime attractors or generators and can include, for example, grocery stores, gas stations, or schools that often define the behavior setting for criminal events (Hart and Miethe 2015). Like with the data representing the user's topic of interest, data files containing the risk-factor information must be a shapefile, KML/KMZ file, or comma delineated (.csv) file with spatial information or address information that can be geocoded.

Despite the growth in its popularity, RTM has some limitations that can restrict its utility as predictive policing tool. For example, RTM uses Kernel Density Estimation (KDE) to produce its prospective maps; but as was described in the previous section, several user-defined parameters must be established prior to running KDE that can affect output (see Fig. 5.3). These settings can include (1) the type of estimation technique to use (e.g., single versus duel KDE), (2) the method for interpolation (e.g., the kernel function), (3) the bandwidth (e.g., the size of the search radius used by the kernel), and (4) the output format units (e.g., grid cell size) in which the KDE results will be generated. Although the RTM tool conducts analysis to determine optimal settings for some of these parameters, others are not and this limitation could lead to unreliable results.

RTM users are also responsible for deciding which "risk-factor layers" should be included and excluded in the modeling of the environmental backcloth of the study area. This decision is supposed to be informed by research, theory, and "intuition" but is open to a degree of subjectivity that could have a substantial impact of the final prospective maps. For example, if every risk factor available for analysis is added to a RTM model, spurious correlations will emerge simple due to the number of variables in the model.

Finally, in most study areas, the interpolated maps produced by RTM will almost entirely consist of "no risk" cells (i.e., grid cells with raster values equal to zero) and cells with values that are nonsense (i.e., risk values over lakes, rivers, or highways) and the spatial relationships observed in the output between cells often produce significant values that are inaccurate due to spatial autocorrelation. Collectively, these shortcomings of RTM limit its applicability as a reliable predictive analytic tool.

5.4 Predictive Policing Methods

The use of predictive policing algorithms to forecast crime represents a shift away from retrospective and prospective mapping techniques described previously. It is a new approach aimed at locating patterns in crime data that identify criminal activity in the near future. These patterns can be exploited directly to prevent crime (i.e. inform resource allocation) and is a distinct approach from how crime analysis has historically been conducted; it prioritizes recent events over distant ones and applies dynamic algorithms to identify spatiotemporal patterns in data.

5.4.1 Commercial Products

Two commercial vendors dominate the current predictive policing software market: PredPol and Azavea. PredPol bills itself as "The Predictive Policing Company" and claims its software is more than just a hot spot tool. PredPol's software analyses "criminal behavior patterns" together with three data points: "past type, place and time of crime" to provide "law enforcement agency with customized crime predictions for the places and times that crimes are most likely to occur" (PredPol 2018). PredPol's prediction algorithms are derived from the field of seismology (i.e., self-exciting point process modeling) and models are updated with new crime data every six months to allow them to produce more accurate forecast.

Law enforcement agencies in Los Angeles, California; Hagerstown, Maryland; and Orange County, Florida have used PredPol reportedly to reduce crime in each of their jurisdictions.

Working with academics from Rutgers University and Temple University, software development company Azavea has created another popular software product used in predictive policing: HunchLab. Law enforcement agencies feed the HunchLab algorithm with cartographic data, including data that defines an agency's jurisdiction, divisions, and beats; they also provide data such as calls for service or crime location information. HunchLab then processes that information to produce prospective crime hot spot maps to be used by law enforcement agencies—similar to those produced from RTM methods—for targeted crime prevention efforts. HunchLab is used in Philadelphia, Pennsylvania and Miami, Florida; and is being tested by the New York Police Department.

5.4.2 PROVE

PROVE is a non-commercial predictive policing software application that was recently developed by researchers at Temple University. Similar to commercial products like PredPol and HunchLab, PROVE uses past crime event information, combined with long-term crime indicators, to model the likelihood of future crime. This information is used to create prospective crime forecasts that, according to the developers, "enables police departments and other agencies across the country to use geocoded crime data in combination with freely available census data to create micro-spatial estimates of future criminal activity at the local level. The output of the utility is a simple map of statistically significant areas of high risk" (Hunchlab 2018). Figure 5.5 shows an example of micro-spatial estimates of future criminal activity at the local level.

A number of research studies have been undertaken in the field of predictive policing using many of the products and algorithms discussed above. Predictive policing analytics, and in particular prospective mapping, have been shown to produce significant reductions in crime. In one of the most robust evaluation to date, Mohler et al. (2015) demonstrated an average 7.4% reduction in multiple crime types (burglary, car theft, theft from vehicle) as a result of directing patrols to areas identified as being at an increased risk based on a predictive algorithm that incorporates both short and long-term crime trends. In more targeted applications reductions, as large as 26% (in residential burglary) have been observed as a result of adopting predictive policing practices (Fielding and Jones 2012).

Despite these promising results, the National Academies of Sciences' Committee on Proactive Policing recently concluded that "there are insufficient robust empirical studies to draw any firm conclusion about either the efficacy of crime-prediction software or the effectiveness of any associated police operational tactics. Furthermore, it is as yet unclear whether predictive policing is substantively different from hot spots policing" (Weisburd and Majmundar 2018, p. 132).

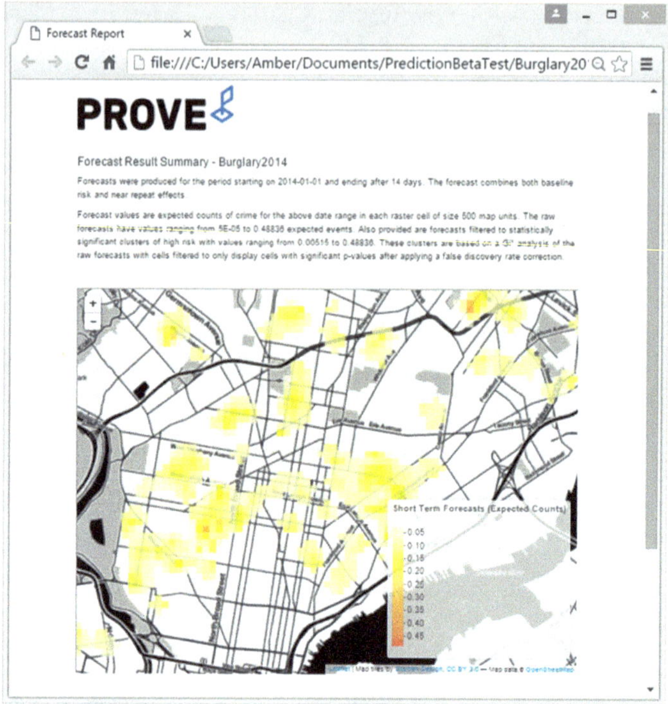

Fig. 5.5 PROVE utility output showing a map of statistically significant areas of high risk of criminal victimization

5.5 Conclusions

Crime hot spot mapping can take three primary forms: retrospective techniques, prospective methods, and complex prediction algorithms. Crime hot spot mapping allows analysts and researchers to identify spatio-temporal patterns in crime data and is often used to identify and propose solutions for criminal offenses, monitor the effectiveness of crime intervention strategies, or to assist in the deployment and management of police operations. More advanced crime mapping techniques allow researchers and agency personnel to move beyond the identification of individual crime locations to a deeper analysis of crime trends and patterns. Interest in crime mapping is growing, as more and more agencies express adopt this technology and researchers continue to develop and test more advanced methods for identifying patterns in data. In many ways, the field of crime mapping can be considered to be in its infancy.

References

Anselin, L. (1995). Local indicators of spatial association–LISA. *Geographical Analysis, 27*(2), 93–115.

Bailey, T., & Gatrell, A. (1995). *Interactive spatial data analysis*. Essex, England: Longman Scientific and Technical.

Ball, G. H., & Hall, D. J. (1970). A clustering technique for summarizing multivariate data. *Behavioral Science, 12,* 153–155.

Barnum, J. D., Caplan, J. M., Kennedy, L. W., & Piza, E. L. (2017). The crime kaleidoscope: A cross-jurisdictional analysis of place features and crime in three urban environments. *Applied Geography, 79,* 203–211. https://doi.org/10.1016/j.apgeog.2016.12.011.

Bates, S. (1987). *Spatial and temporal analysis of crime. Research bulletin, April, 1987*. Chicago: Illinois Criminal Justice Information Authority.

Birks, D., Townsley, M., & Hart, T. C. (2019). *Predictive policing in an Australian context: Assessing viability and utility*. Australia Institute of Criminology (AIC): Canberra, Australia.

Bowers, K. J., Johnson, S. D., & Pease, K. (2004). Prospective hot-spotting: The future of crime mapping? *British Journal of Criminology, 44,* 641–658.

Brantingham, P. J. (2018). The logic of data bias and its impact on place-based predictive policing. *Ohio State Journal of Criminal Law, 15,* 473–486.

Brunsdon, C. (1995). Estimating probability surfaces for geographical point data: An adaptive kernel algorithm. *Computers & Geosciences, 21*(7), 877–894.

Canter, P. (1993). Hot spot area analysis in Baltimore County. *STACNews* (vol.1) (Winter, 1993).

Caplan, J. M., & Kennedy, L. W. (2010). *Risk terrain modeling manual: Theoretical framework and technical steps of spatial risk assessment*. Newark, NJ: Rutgers Center on Public Security.

Caplan, J. M., Kennedy, L. W., & Miller, J. (2011). Risk terrain modeling: Brokering criminological theory and GIS methods for crime forecasting. *Justice Quarterly, 28*(2), 360–381.

Caplan, J. M., Kennedy, L. W., & Piza, E. L. (2013). Joint utility of event-dependent and environmental crime analysis techniques for violent crime forecasting. *Crime & Delinquency, 59*(2), 243–270. https://journals.sagepub.com/doi/abs/10.1177/0011128712461901.

Chainey, S., & Ratcliffe, J. H. (2005). *GIS and crime mapping*. San Francisco, CA: Wiley.

Chainey, S., Tompson, L., & Uhlig, S. (2008a). The utility of hotspot mapping for predicting patterns of crime. *Security Journal, 21,* 4–28.

Chainey, S., Tompson, L., & Uhlig, S. (2008b). Response to Pezzuchi. *Security Journal, 21,* 293–294.

Chainey, S., Tompson, L., & Uhlig, S. (2008c). Response to Levine. *Security Journal, 21,* 303–306.

D'Andrade, R. (1978). U-statistic hierarchical clustering. *Psychometrika, 4,* 58–67.

Drawve, G., & Barnum, J. D. (2015). Place-based risk factors for aggravated assault across police divisions in Little Rock, Arkansas. *Journal of Crime and Justice, 41*(2), 173–192.

Eck, J. E., Chainey, S., Cameron, J. G., Leitner, M., & Wilson, R. E. (2005). *Mapping crime: Understanding hotspots*. National Institute of Justice Special Report.

Edmonds, W., & Mallard, J. (2011, September). *Using risk terrain modeling to analyze holiday robberies in Arlington, TX*. Paper presented at the training conference of the International Association of Crime Analysts, Hyannis, MA.

Fielding, M., & Jones, V. (2012). Disrupting the optimal forager: Predictive risk mapping and domestic burglary reduction in Trafford, Greater Manchester. *International Journal of Police Science & Management, 14*(1), 30–41.

Garnier, S., Caplan, J. M., & Kennedy, L. W. (2018). Predicting dynamical crime distribution from environmental and social influences. *Frontiers in Applied Mathematics and Statistics*. Online first at https://doi.org/10.3389/fams.2018.00013.

Getis, A., & Ord, J. K. (1992). The analysis of spatial association by use of distance statistics. *Geographical Analysis, 24*(3), 189–206.

Groff, E. R., & Taniguchi, T. (2018). *Micro-level policing for preventing near repeat residential burglary: Final monograph*. Washington, D.C.: Police Foundation.
Hart, T. C., & Miethe, T. D. (2015). Configural behavior settings of crime event locations: Towards an alternative conceptualization of criminogenic micro-environments. *Journal of Research in Crime and Delinquency, 52*(3), 373–402. https://doi.org/10.1177/0022427814566639.
Hart, T. C., & Zandbergen, P. A. (2012). *Effects of data quality on predictive hotspot mapping* (NCJ-239861). Final technical report prepared for the National Institute of Justice in compliance with cooperative agreement #2009-IJ-CX-0022. Washington, D.C.
Hart, T. C., & Zandbergen, P. A. (2013). Reference data and geocoding quality: Examining completeness and positional accuracy of street geocoded crime incidents. *Policing: An International Journal of Police Strategies & Management, 36*(2), 263–294.
Hart, T. C., & Zandbergen, P. A. (2014). Kernel density estimation and hotspot mapping: Examining the influence of interpolation method, grid cell size, and bandwidth on crime forecasting. *Policing: An International Journal of Police Strategies & Management, 37*(2), 305–323.
Hartigan, J. A. (1975). *Clustering algorithms*. New York: Wiley.
Hunchlab. (2018). *PROVE utility* [Apparatus and software]. Azavea. Philadelphia, PA.
Johnson, S. C. (1967). Hierarchical clustering schemes. *Psychometrika, 32,* 241–254.
Johnson, S. D., & Bowers, K. J. (2004). The stability of space-time clusters of burglary. *The British Journal of Criminology, 44*(1), 55–65.
Johnson, S. D., Summers, L., & Pease, K. (2009). Offender as forager? A direct test of the boost account of victimization. *Journal of Quantitative Criminology, 25*(2), 181–200.
Levine, N. (2008). The "hottest" part of a hotspot: Comments on "The utility of hotspot mapping for predicting spatial patters of crime". *Security Journal, 21,* 295–302.
Levine, N. (2015). *CrimeStat: A spatial statistics program for the analysis of crime incident locations* (v 4.02) [Apparatus and software]. Ned Levine & Associates, Houston, Texas, and the National Institute of Justice, Washington, D.C.
McBratney, A. B., & deBruijter, J. J. (1992). A continuum approach to soil classification by modified fuzzy k-means with extragrades. *Journal of Soil Science, 43,* 159–175.
Mohler, G. O., Short, M. B., Malinowski, S., Johnson, M., Tita, G. E., Bertozzi, A. L., et al. (2015). Randomized control field trials of predictive policing. *Journal of the American Statistical Association, 110*(512), 1399–1411. https://doi.org/10.1080/01621459.2015.1077710.
Ord, J. K., & Getis, A. (1995). Local spatial autocorrelation statistics: Distributional issues and an application. *Geographical Analysis, 27*(4), 286–306.
Perry, W. L., McInnis, B., Price, C. C., Smith, S. C., & Hollywood, J. S. (2013). *Predictive policing: The role of crime forecasting in law enforcement operations*. Washington, D.C.: Rand Corporation.
Pezzuchi, G. (2008). A brief commentary on "The utility of hotspot mapping for predicting spatial patterns of crime". *Security Journal, 21,* 291–292.
Piza, E. L., Kennedy, L. W., & Caplan, J. M. (2018). Facilitators and impediments to designing, implementing, and evaluating risk-based policing strategies using risk terrain modeling: Insights from a multi-city evaluation in the United States. *European Journal of Criminal Policy and Research, 24*(4), 489–513. https://doi.org/10.1007/s10610-017-9367-9.
Predpol. (2018). How PredPol works: We provide guidance on where and when to patrol. Retrieved from http://www.predpol.com/how-predpol-works/ (Accessed June 3, 2018).
Ratcliffe, J. H. (2007). *Near repeat calculator* [Apparatus and software]. Philadelphia, PA: Temple University. Retrieved from http://www.cla.temple.edu/cj/resources/near-repeat-calculator/ (Accessed June 3, 2018).
Ratcliffe, J. H. (2014). What is the future…of predictive policing? *Translational Criminology, 6,* 4–5.
Ratcliffe, J. H., & Rengert, G. F. (2008). Near-repeat patterns in Philadelphia shootings. *Security Journal, 21,* 58–76.

Short, M. B., D'Orsogna, M. R., Brantingham, P. J., & Tita, G. E. (2009). Measuring and modeling repeat and near-repeat burglary effects. *Journal of Quantitative Criminology, 25*(3), 325–339. https://doi.org/10.1007/s10940-009-9068-8.

Spring, J. V., & Block, C. R. (1989). *STAC user's manual*. Chicago: Illinois Criminal Justice Information Authority.

Tseloni, A., & Pease, K. (2003). Repeat personal victimization. 'Boosts' or 'flags'? *The British Journal of Criminology, 43*(1), 196–212.

Thompson, H. R. (1956). Distribution of distance to nth neighbour in a population of randomly distributed individuals. *Ecology, 37,* 391–394.

Townsley, M., Homel, R., & Chaseling, J. (2003). Infectious burglaries: A test of the near repeat hypothesis. *The British Journal of Criminology, 43*(1), 615–633.

Ward, J. H. (1963). Hierarchical grouping to optimize an objective function. *Journal of the American Statistical Association, 58,* 236–244.

Weisburd, D., & Majmundar, M. K. (2018). *Proactive policing: Effects on crime and communities*. Washington, D.C.: National Academies Press.

Yerxa, M. (2013). Evaluating the temporal parameters of risk terrain modeling with residential burglary. *Crime Mapping: A Journal of Research and Practice, 5*(1), 7–38.

Chapter 6
Geographic Variations in, and Correlates of Green/Environmental Crime Across US States: A Preliminary Assessment

Michael J. Lynch, Michael A. Long and Paul B. Stretesky

The study of green crimes was first introduced into criminology thirty years ago (Lynch 1990). Green crimes are behaviors that generate two types of harms. First, they harm ecosystems either locally or globally through behaviors such as pollution, or through ecological resource extraction. Environmental sociology, which is the origin of these terms, refer to these adverse behaviors as ecological additions and ecological withdrawals respectively. Second, ecological additions and withdrawals not only produce primary or direct harms, they also generate secondary or indirect harms. Those indirect harms may affect other portions of the ecosystem, or living beings. These living beings included Gaia (the living earth system), human beings, and all nonhuman beings (which could be divided into categories such as wildlife, or nonhuman animals, or nonhuman mammals, or birds, or fish, or trees and plants, etc.,). To examine these outcomes, green criminology also includes the study of laws and forms of social control that relate to green crime, as well as the study of environmental justice broadly conceived.

One criticisms levied against green criminology is that it contains relatively few quantitative studies, especially those that assess hypotheses, and is empirically deficient in comparison to other portions of the criminological literature (Lynch et al. 2017a, b; Lynch and Pires 2019). Employing a generous (i.e., broad) definition of both the term empirical and green criminology (following Lynch and Pires (2019), which also included studies in conservation criminology), there were fewer

M. J. Lynch (✉)
Department of Criminology, University of South Florida, Tampa, USA
e-mail: mjlynch@usf.edu

M. A. Long
Department of Sociology, Oklahoma State University, Stillwater, USA
e-mail: michael.long@okstate.edu

P. B. Stretesky
Department of Social Sciences, Northumbria University, Newcastle upon Tyne, UK
e-mail: PAUL.STRETESKY@NORTHUMBRIA.AC.UK

K. M. Lersch and J. Chakraborty (eds.), *Geographies of Behavioural Health, Crime, and Disorder*, GeoJournal Library 126,
https://doi.org/10.1007/978-3-030-33467-3_6

than 120 empirical studies published in these areas from 1998 to 2018—or only 6 per year on average. Given that small body of empirical literature, there are core or key green criminological questions that have yet to be examined. Neglecting those core/key questions means some very basic knowledge concerning the extent and distribution of green crimes remains unknown.

The present study examined some of those core questions by exploring the geographic distribution of green crimes across US states. It is based on three observations about the study of street and green crime. First, the geographic distribution of street crime has long been studied. Numerous criminological studies examine the geography of street crime at different levels of analysis, including across states, in an effort to determine whether the distribution of crime might yield some information that might help explain and control crime. Research indicating persistent geographic crime patterns are among the most robust and oldest empirical findings in criminology. Based on these persistent findings, one could assume that green/environmental crime might also have a geographic distribution that could, for example, vary across US states. This possibility has yet to be sufficiently explored, and little is known about the geography of green crime.

Second, the geographic study of street crime has also produced social and economic correlates of crime. There is, however, no comparable literature on the geographic correlates of green crime. Given the omission of such studies, we do not know, for example, whether the correlates of street crime are also associated with the distribution of green crimes. Moreover, given differences in the nature of street and green crimes, there may be unique correlates of green crime. But, because those correlates have not been sufficiently explored, there is little relevant information about the correlates of green crimes.

Third, and not surprisingly given the above, prior studies have not examined whether green crimes and street crimes have similar distributions. While criminologists have employed cross-state data to assess factors that influence street crime levels and distributions (e.g. Allan and Steffensmeier 1989; Chamlin and Cochran 1997, 1995; Chintrakarn and Herzer 2012; Kawachi et al. 1999; Land et al. 1990; Quinney 1966; Raphael and Winter-Ebmer 2001; Rosenfeld et al. 2005), such studies have not been undertaken with environmental crime data. In addition, studies have not examined whether different measures of green crime are related across geographic locations.

In the absence of prior studies on these issues, one might hypothesize that the distribution of environmental offenses are a product of differences in environmental enforcement across states, including the number of state agencies charged with enforcing environmental laws and environmental protection budgets. This hypothesis, which suggest that crime data has a relationship to the organization of social control and the organization of agencies that both control crime and record crime statistics, has been well recognized for forty years in the criminological literature (McCleary et al. 1982). In addition, it is possible that other state characteristics such as population density, manufacturing concentration or other measures of economic processes, state land use patterns, urbanization, and demographic characteristics may impact variability in environmental crimes across states.

A number of these correlates were examined for this research. The criminological literature, however, has not assessed whether any of these factors correlate with green/environmental crime across states.

The present study addresses ***cross-state variation*** in environmental violations at US EPA registered facilities. The offenses examine included violations of the Clean Air Act (CAA), Clean Water Act (CWA), and Resource Conservation and Recovery Act (RCRA) and Toxic Release Inventory (TRI). Employing these data, we assess variations in, and potential correlates of: (1) the number and rate of current environmental violations at facilities (2015); (2) the number and rate of three year continuing environmental violations at facilities (2013–2015); (3) the number and rate of formal environmental enforcement actions (2011–2015); (4) whether the geographic distribution of green and street crimes overlap across states; and (5) search for correlates related to the geography of green crime.

6.1 Prior Research

The study of green/environmental crimes emerged as an area of criminological research in 1990 (Lynch 1990). That literature is now diverse, and has examined a wide range of issues including: non-human animal abuse (Beirne 1999); bio-piracy (Goyes and South 2015); food crimes (Walters 2007); toxic victimization from corporate environmental crimes (Lynch and Stretesky 2001); deforestation crimes (van Solinge 2010); the generation of green crimes by the treadmill of production (Stretesky et al. 2013; Lynch et al. 2013); green-cultural criminology (Brisman and South 2013). This body of research also includes a growing number of empirical studies examining animal poaching (Petrossian and Clarke 2013; Petrossian et al. 2015; Pires and Clarke 2011, 2012), wildlife trade (Stretesky et al. 2018), environmental justice (Stretesky and Lynch 1998, 1999, 2002), factors predicting environmental law violations (Lynch et al. 2004a, b; Stretesky and Lynch 2011), and the formal (Stretesky and Lynch 2009) and informal enforcement of environmental regulations (Lynch and Stretesky 2013). Much of the green criminological literature is theoretical, or built around case studies. A significant limitation of that literature is a lack of quantitative studies (Lynch et al. 2017a, b), and there are few empirical studies examining the geographic distribution of green crime across US states (Lynch et al. 2017a, b). Thus, despite the growth of this literature, little is known about the distribution of environmental/green crime across place or time.

Within the US, prior studies on the distribution of environmental crime are limited and dated. Most are temporal rather than geographic (Cohen 1992; Lynch 2017; Lynch et al. 2016; McMurray and Ramsey 1986; O'Hear 2004). In geographic terms, existing empirical studies tend to focus on single states, ignoring variations and concentrations of green crimes across place (Crow et al. 2013). Cross-state studies have also focused on green crime as an environmental justice concern (Stretesky and Lynch 2011) rather than strictly exploring the geography of green crime more generally.

6.2 Data

Data for this study were drawn from a variety of sources, and are detailed where necessary. The dependent variables were drawn from the US Environmental Protection Agency's *Environmental Compliance History Online* database (ECHO; http://echo.epa.gov), and included: (1) current environmental offenses; (2) three-year noncompliance offenses; and (3) five-year formal enforcement actions. These indicators measure aggregated environmental violations for the Clean Water Act (CWA), Clean Air Act (CAA), Resource Conservation Recovery Act (RCRA), and Toxic Release Inventory (TRI) for each US state. The data measure violations by US EPA registered facilities in each state.

We examined the data at the state level. Since, as noted, there have been no prior studies of the distribution of green crimes or their relationship to street crimes, it makes sense to begin with a larger unit of analysis where there is also accessible information about the distribution of street crimes. Moreover, since this is a preliminary study, it is useful to examine general hypotheses at a broad level of analysis to determine whether they have any merit. Whether those hypotheses are rejected or not at the macro-level, does not mean they may not have utility at lower levels of aggregation, and future research can be developed to address these issues using disaggregated data.

Current violations (CV) are environmental violations that occurred during the prior year (2015; see below for additional details). Three-year noncompliance (3YNC) measures the persistence of environmental offending by counting a facility's number of quarters in noncompliance over three years (2013–2015). It should be noted that noncompliance offenses *are not* a simple sum of three consecutive years of current violations (CV). When a facility is charged with a current violation, they are also issued conditions for remedying the violation. Facilities that remedy the violation are then removed from the offense data because they are no longer in noncompliance. Thus, noncompliance measures facilities identified as being in noncompliance in 2013, that also failed to remedy an offense through 2015. The five-year count of formal enforcement actions (5EA) is the only measure available from EPA that assess the use of formal punishments for environmental violations. It is the count of formal enforcement actions taken against a facility in the prior five years.

The above variables were used as counts and also transformed into rates. Rate measures *have not* often been employed in the green criminological literature. In contrast, rates are commonly used in the study of street crime to make comparisons over time or place that adjust for population size effects. Street crime rates are typically calculated per 100,000 people. This measure has logical appeal to the extent that people are the violators in street crime, and the number of people in a given location could impact the number of offenses in that location. Since population size could affect the number of street crimes within a geographic area, and because geographic areas may have non-comparable base populations, criminologists often use population based crime rates. In contrast to street crimes, the green crimes measured here are not committed by individuals, though clearly individuals must act for those crimes to occur. Rather, they are counted as being committed by corporations or businesses. Thus, the rate of green crimes were constructed by crime type measure, and standardized per 100 US EPA registered facilities within each state.

ECHO data for this study were collected on December 7th, 2015. We note this date because ECHO is a "rolling" database, updated weekly. Each time the database is refreshed or updated, the time frame covered changes (e.g., when a new week is added, the oldest week is subtracted). Thus, for current offenses, the data covers December 5th, 2014–December 6th, 2015; for three-year noncompliance, December 5th, 2012–December 6th, 2015; and for formal enforcement, December 5th, 2010 to December 6th, 2015.

Given the time-linked nature of the dependent variable, it was not possible to measure all the independent variables for the same time periods. We matched time periods for independent variables as closely as possible to dependent variable time periods. Several independent variables, however, were measured several years before the dependent variables. For some independent variables, these are the only available indicators (i.e., decennial measures); for others, the measurement time period should not change the measurement (e.g., miles of rivers and streams are relatively constant); and for other measures, the differences over short periods of time are negligible (e.g., some physical measures of states, such as percent of land in agricultural production changes slowly). Nevertheless, due to these time-dependent measurement issues, the regression analyses examining potential correlates of environmental crimes should not be employed to make causal inferences.

The green/environmental crime measures are known environmental crimes at US EPA registered facilities. Thus, these data only measure the official distribution of environmental crimes facilities commit, and excludes other types of green/environmental crimes (e.g., those committed by individuals against wildlife, pets/companion animals, farm animals, laboratory animals, etc.,). Consequently, our data should not be taken as an indicator of the full extent of environmental crime across states.

Assessing the distribution of green crimes across states, its relationship to street crimes and the potential geographic correlates of green crimes required examining a great deal of cross-state data. Due to space restrictions, we limited our use of tables, particularly for regression analyses which involved estimating more than three dozen initial models, and often produced no notable significant results. While we describe results using model identifiers throughout the manuscript as a mechanism to keep track of the results (e.g., Model 1), we display a limited number of the most useful models in table form. The results across the various regression estimates are also summarized in table form (see Table 4).

6.3 Variation in Current Offenses, Number and Rate

Across the 50 states, there were 53,655 total current environmental offenses (CEV), which ranged between 98 (Hawaii) to 5485 (Texas), with a mean of 1073.1 per state. Thirty-four states had fewer environmental offenses than the mean, and the distribution was positively skewed (skewness = 2.164; kurtosis = 6.078).

We then transformed the count into the current environmental offense rate (CEVR) per 100 facilities. The rate varied between 0.74/100 (Minnesota) to 29.26/100 (Washington) facilities, with a mean of 8.31. The maximum rate is nearly 40 times the minimum rate. Thirty-one states had rates below the mean, and the distribution was positively skewed (skewness = 1.651; kurtosis = 3.20). Here, standardization reduced skewness. Based on prior research, we suspected that skewness in the distribution of environmental measures was a result of the EPA regions in which states are located. In later analyses, we address this issue by controlling for EPA region.

There is a significant correlation between the number of CEVs and the number of pollution permits across states ($r = 0.675$; $p = 0.000$), but, at the same time, a negative, significant correlation between the CEV rate (CEVR) and EPA permits ($r = -0.319$; $p = 0.024$). In other words, when the count data is employed, the number of permits predicts the total number of violations as being positive. However, when this relationship is measured using rates, the correlation indicates that while states with many permits may have a higher current violation ***counts***, they have a low violations ***rates***. Geographically, this outcome suggests that count and rate maps would look quite different. These differences can be seen by comparing the maps in Fig. 6.1 (current violation rate per 100 facilities) to Fig. 6.2 (current violation counts). In short, and not unexpectedly, standardizing the data affects the distribution of known environmental crimes across states. As additional evidence of this outcome, the Pearson correlation coefficient (r) between the rate (CEVR) and count (CEV) for current violations is only 0.189 ($p = 0.389$), indicating that these two measures are not significantly related and potentially measure different qualities of the distribution of environmental violations across states.

Several states had very low and very high CEVR. Thirteen states had CEVRs less than one-half the mean, and six had a CEVRs of 3 or less (California, Florida, Kansas, Maryland, Minnesota, and Virginia) [1]. At the other end of the spectrum, four states had CEVR rates more than twice the mean (Alaska, 17.23; Idaho, 26.22; Texas, 21.45; Washington, 29.26). These results suggest several possible explanations that require further research. Either: (1) enforcement activities in those states are weak, resulting in low rates of known offending; or (2) industries and facilities in those states are more law-abiding than industries/facilities in other states; or (3) variability in the types of industries across states affects the rate of environmental offending. The distribution of current offenses by number and rate (and for other environmental crime measures) can be found in Appendix.

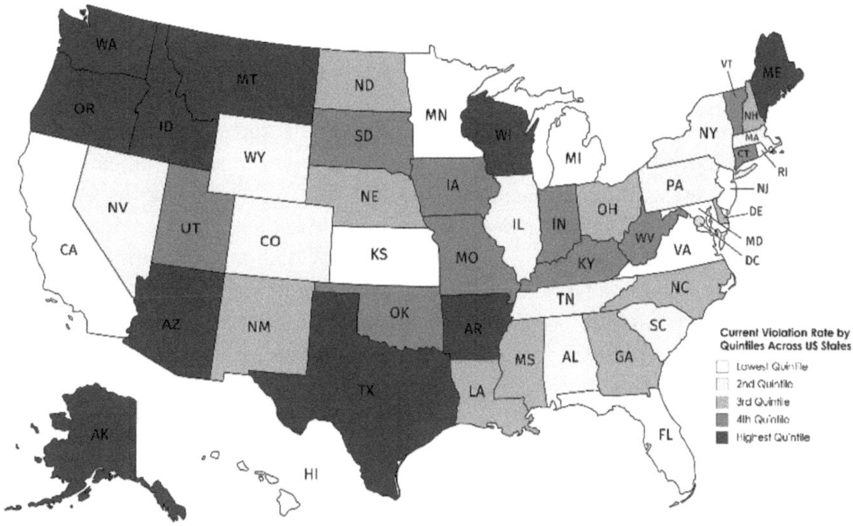

Fig. 6.1 Current violation rate per 100 EPA registered facilities across states shaded by quintile map modeled with http://mapcghart.net

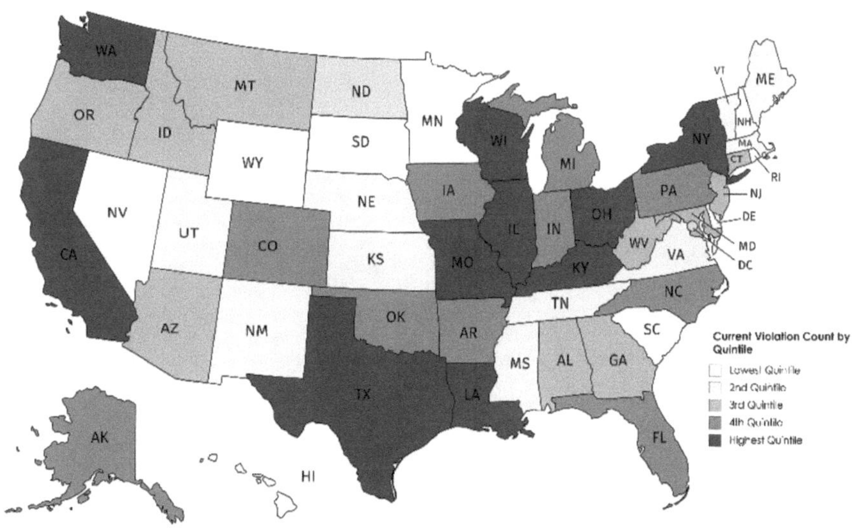

Fig. 6.2 Current violation count data by state shaded by quintile map modeled with http://mapchart.net

6.4 Three Year Facility Noncompliance, Number and Rate

The second indicator of environmental violations is three-year noncompliance (3YNC), which measures noncompliance with environmental obligations and non-remedied Final Order obligations (see Fig. 6.3 for map). Consequently, the 3YNC indicator is not simply a sum of violations over three years since facilities that remedy a Final Order obligation still have a violation, but are no longer in noncompliance. Thus 3YNC measures continuing violations. Despite these differences, the current violation and three year violation distribution across states is highly correlated ($r = 0.897$; $p = 0.000$), indicating that states with large numbers of current violations would be expected to have a large number of continuing violations, which is an important, geographically stable dimension of green crime.

The 3YNC measure ranged from 298 (Hawaii) to 9026 (Texas). States with the fewest and largest number of 3YNC and CEVs were identical. The three year noncompliance mean was 2679, with 33 states below the mean, and a positively skewed distribution (skewness = 1.421; kurtosis = 2.046).

3YNC was also converted into a rate (3YNCR) per 100 regulated facilities, and varied between 5.67 and 58.39. Like the CEVR, 3YNC was lowest in Minnesota and highest in Washington. The mean rate was 21.37, and 33 states were below the mean, indicating a slight positively skewed distribution (skewness = 1.019; kurtosis = 0.855; see Appendix).

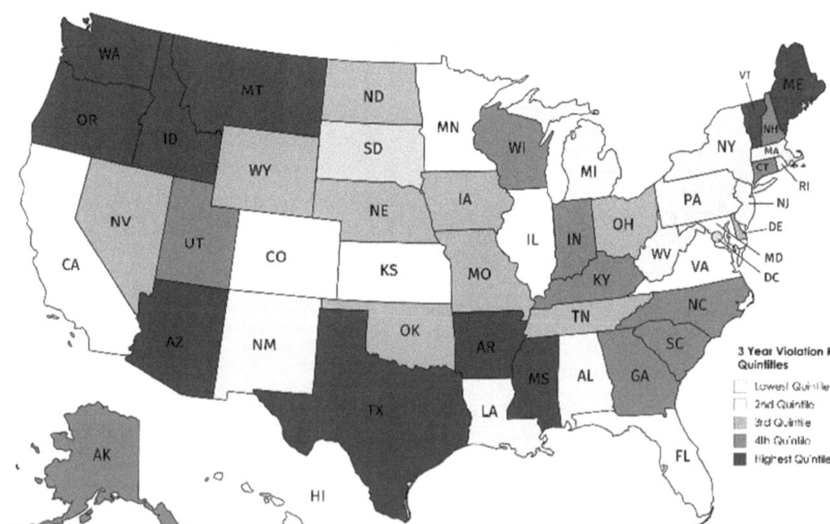

Fig. 6.3 Three year violation rates per 100 EPA facilities across states shaded by quintiles map modeled with http://mapchart.net

The above indicates that the geographic picture of green crime is similar when comparing the count of current violations to the count of continuing violations across states, and also when comparing the rate of current violations and the rate of continuing violations. However the count distributions and the rate distributions are geographically distinct.

6.5 The Overlap Between Environmental Offenses and Street Crimes

The brief analysis above indicates variation in the geographic distribution of environmental crimes across states. It is well known that the distribution of street crime, which tends to be the primary focus of criminological research, also varies across states (see Fig. 6.4). Prior research has yet to examine whether the distribution of green and street crimes are similar or unique.

The distributions of street and green crimes would be hypothesized *to be similar if* the causes of those crimes are comparable. It could also be hypothesized that states with high levels of street crime may be more concerned with controlling crime, which might extend to efforts to control green crime. In contrast, it is also plausible that states with high street crime levels may focus so much attention on that issue, that other kinds of crimes escape their attention; or that states with high levels of street crime might have low levels of green crime if crime control reflects how different forms of law and social control contribute to reinforcing the structural

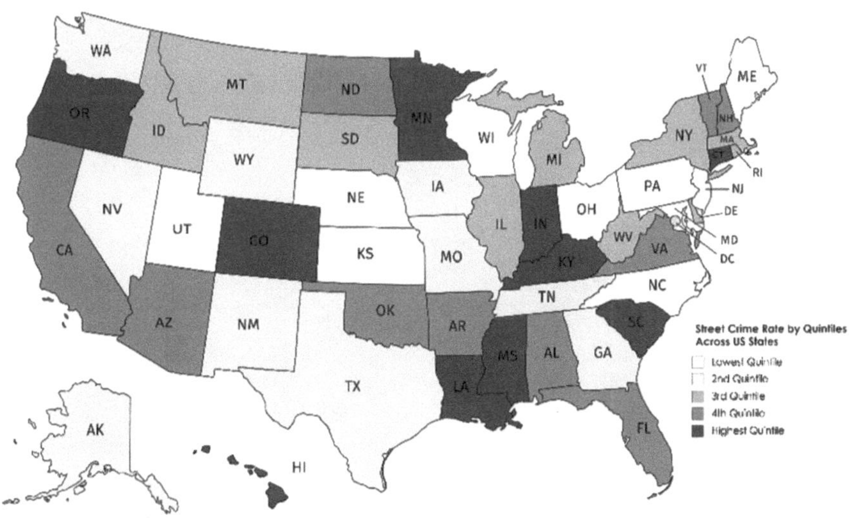

Fig. 6.4 Crime rate per 100,000 population across states shaded by quintile map modeled with http://mapchart.net

dynamics of power in society as suggested by Reiman (1979). Currently, there is no empirical evidence that can address these hypotheses.

A simple test of the above examines the correlations between street and environmental crime rates across states. Street crime rates per 100,000 population were measured using the FBI Uniform Crime Index (UCR) data on crimes known to police. Both the FBI UCR and the EPA ECHO offenses are measures of known offending. The correlation between the index crime rate and CEVR ($r = -0.088$, $p = 0.543$) indicates these rates are unrelated geographically. The outcome is similar for index crime rates and 3YNCR ($r = -0.119$; $p = 0.411$), and these data suggest the geography of street and green crimes are not related. It could be argued that these findings are not surprising since street crimes generally involve enforcement in low income communities against low income offenders, and green crimes generally involve powerful, wealthy offenders.

To explore these findings further, we regressed rates of known UCR violent and property crimes rates against environmental crime (both CEVR and 3YNCR) controlling for EPA region to assess whether variability in environmental crime rates may be related to organizational differences in responses to crime, or perhaps to regional variability. There are ten US EPA regions, and since each region represents a geographic cluster of states, an EPA region affect may represent something unknown about the geographic clustering of states in each region that affects environmental crime (for map of EPA regions see Fig. 6.5).

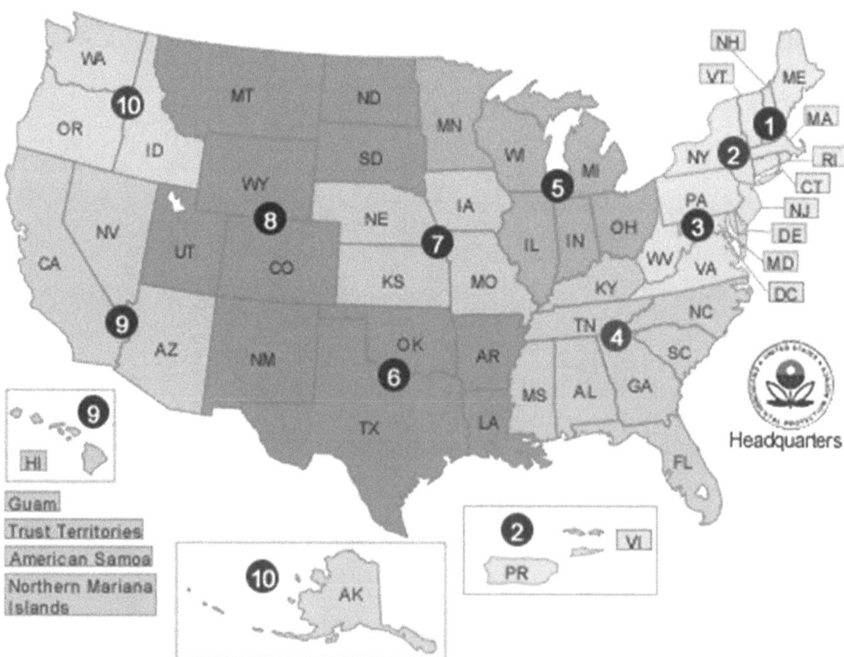

Fig. 6.5 US EPA regions map. *Source* US EPA, regional office map; gray scale edit

In Model 1 (CEVR is the dependent variable), Region 10, which has the highest CEVR/100 facilities, was used as the reference category, and thus the effects for the remaining regions should be negative in the regression model if region plays a significant role. As expected, all included region effects were negative, but also significant ($p = 0.000$). The UCR violent and property crime rates were insignificant, however (Adj. $R^2 = 0.433$; VIFs for all variables less than 2.7). Model 1 indicated that CEVR was related to EPA regions, but that the level of street crime was not, suggesting that perhaps CEVR across states has some organizational or regional component.

In Model 2 (3YNCR), Region 10 was again employed as the omitted comparison category. As expected, all included regions had a negative relationship to the dependent variable, and again, all were statistically significant ($p = 0.015$ or less). Controlling for EPA region, the UCR property crime rate was statistically insignificant, while the UCR *violent crime rate was statistically significant and negative* ($p = 0.018$). Thus, as the violent crime rate increased, 3YNCR decreased, an outcome consistent with the class control model (Adj. $R^2 = 0.347$; all VIFs below 2.698)—that is, as the control of street crime increased, the control of green crime declined. Additional analysis found no effect for the aggregated (property plus violent) crime rate on environmental crime types across states.

Looking across these outcomes, these results suggest street crime and green crime rates are unrelated across states. Where they were related (violent crime and 3YNCR), the relationship was inverse, and supported a class-control hypothesis. Why violent crime is inversely related to the three year and not the current rate of green crime, however, is somewhat of a mystery.

These results showed a persistent EPA region effect. That outcome suggests a possible organizational crime control effect, or some other unmeasured state level or regional effect. To assess whether the geographic distribution might be influenced by state level environmental organizational factors, we re-estimated the above equations (Models 1 and 2) adding various state-level environmental agency indicators (e.g., number of agencies, gross spending, per capita spending). These variables did not produce any statistically significant effects.

6.6 Five Year Formal Enforcement, Numbers and Rates

In theory, one would expect that the volume of environmental offenses is related to environmental enforcement. One might expect that states with more environmental violations might also have a more formal enforcement actions, and that the geographic distribution of these two outcomes would be related. In the US EPA ECHO data, enforcement is measured by a five year indicator of formal enforcement actions (5EA) described earlier (a map for the distribution of enforcement is found in Fig. 6.6).

The number of 5EA across states varies from a low of 14 (South Dakota) to a high of 3467 (North Carolina), with a mean of 663.08. It should be kept in mind

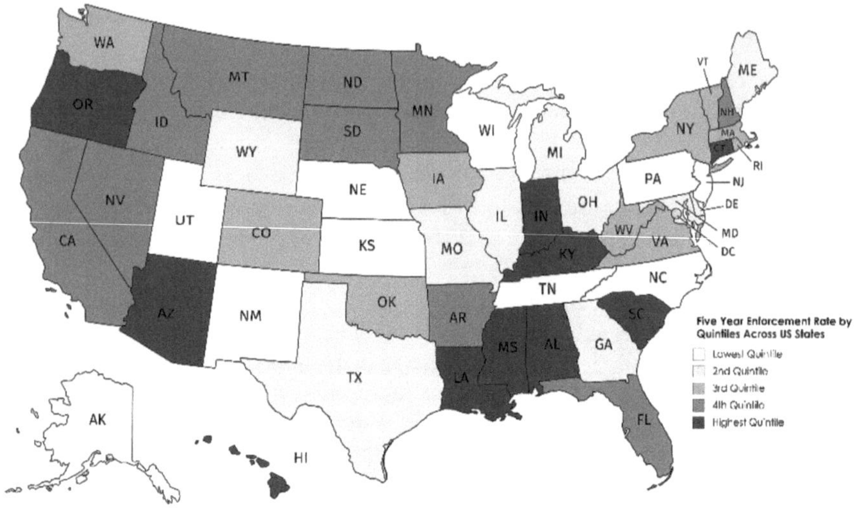

Fig. 6.6 Five year enforcement rate per 100 EPA registered facilities across states shaded by quintiles map modeled with http://mapcghart.net

that these are five-year and not annual means. The distribution is highly skewed with 38 states below the mean (skewness = 2.130; kurtosis = 4.730).

We used the 5EA count data to create two environmental enforcement rates: E-Rate1 and E-Rate2. E-Rate1 (ER1) is the enforcement rate per 100 facilities, calculated by dividing the number of formal enforcement actions by the number of EPA permitted (CWA, CAA, RCRA) and reporting (TRI) facilities in each state, multiplied by 100. ER1 is a fairly traditional enforcement rate measure estimating offending rates against potential offenders (in this case is facilities). Because the denominator is facilities, ER1 can be compared to the previously described environmental violation rates that also employed a facility denominator. One must keep in mind, however, that ER1, is calculated over a 5 year period, and so it could be substantially larger than the comparable environmental violation rates which can only be measured as one- and three-year offending rates. The range for ER1 is 0.76/100 facilities (North Dakota) to 19.65 (North Carolina), with a mean of 4.26 (skewness = 2.996; kurtosis = 14.131). ER1 data indicates that punishment is relative rare for environmental offenses. Thirty-five states have ER1 of 5/100 or less, and North Carolina is the only state with an ER1 greater than 10/100.

E-Rate2 (ER2) is a punishment rate for formal environmental enforcement relative to the volume of offending over five years. It was measured as the ratio of the rate of environmental enforcement to the rate of three year noncompliance. A measure of 1.0 indicates that ER2 is equivalent to 3YNCR, meaning that all cases potentially eligible for punishment receive a formal penalty response. Because the denominator is a three-year rate, and the numerator is a five year rate, *ER2 overestimates* the likelihood that an environmental violation yields a formal punishment response. Despite its limitation, this is the best available measure of this rate because of the way the environmental punishment and offending data is maintained by US EPA. The range for ER2 was 0.02 (Vermont) to 0.93 (North Carolina), and had a mean of 0.243, with 29 states below the mean (skewness = 1.892; kurtosis = 4.821). The mean indicates that 24.3% of violations result in a formal punishment. Moreover, since the denominator, 3YNCR, is a measure of non-remediated offending, and the count and rate of 3YNCR is lower than the three year sum of current violations would be (CEV), the punishment rate yielded by the ER2 procedure is likely much higher than a single year punishment rate would be (which cannot be calculated given the way the data are maintained).

ER1 and ER2 are highly correlated (r = 0.698, p = 0.000), but the correlation also suggests each indicator measures some unique aspect of the distribution of environmental punishment. We also ran correlations between the punishment/enforcement rates, and the offense rates for green crimes as a preliminary examination of potential associations. The correlations between ER1 and CEVR (0.162) and 3NCYR (0.203) were fairly low. The correlations between ER2 and CEVR and 3NCYR were substantially higher, but negative (−0.397 and −0.464). Interestingly, these results indicate that the five-year punishment rate adjusting for facilities, and the current and three-year offending rates are only weakly related. In an additional regression analysis, controlling for other predictors, the impact of offending on punishment was insignificant. In contrast, the five-year punishment rate adjusted for offending was more strongly correlated with the current and three-year offending rates. This should be expected since here, the correlated measures share a dimension. However, for ER2, the negative relationship clearly indicates that the distribution of punishment and offending is inversely related, so that punishment is more likely where there are fewer offenders.

6.7 Summary: Cross-State Variability in Environmental Crimes

Our initial assessment discovered significant variability in the reported/known volume of environmental offending and punishment across states. Current violations (CEV) over the past year ranged from 98 to 5485. That difference is due, in part, to the number of potential violators, which was controlled by converting CEV into a rate (CEVR). Across states, the number of potential violators ranged from 1821 (Delaware) to 60,040 (California). Accounting for facilities, CEVR ranged from 0.74 to 29.26, with a mean of 8.31. Both measures indicate large variability in the volume of known environmental offenses across states, but relatively low offense rates. In comparison, the mean number of street crimes across states in 2015, was about 2800 per 100,000, which is equivalent to about 2.8/100. *As a measure of the concentration of crime, the rate of green crimes* (8.31) *is almost three times higher than the concentration of street crimes.* For the traditional criminologist concerned with street crime, this result is unexpected; the incidence rate of green crime is much higher than the incidence rate for street crime. Little attention has been paid to this empirical reality of crime, and the criminological literature remains focused on street crime. While the terms "street crime" and "green crime" are not used exclusively in the criminological literature, searching those terms in google scholar provides some idea of the difference in the quantity of research focused on each area. Using google scholar, and limiting the search to 2017, the term "street crime" appears 1620 times, which is 24.2 times more often than the term "green crime" appeared in the published literature.

The three year indicator of noncompliance (3NC) also suggests significant variability in known environmental offending by facilities across states. The 3YNC range was 298–9026 cases, and for the rate data, 5.67–58.39 per 100 facilities. Here, again, accounting for facility concentration by calculating offending rates significantly reduced variability in the scope of noncompliance.

The data also indicated large variations in formal responses to environmental violations across states. As a count, 5EA ranged from 14 to 3467, but as a rate/100 facilities varied from 0.76 to 19.65. Despite the fact that the 5EA rate measures punishments over five years, it is significantly lower than the offending rates, indicating that across states, punishment for these offenses is rare. The ER2 measure for environmental punishment also indicated wide variability (N = 2–93) in environmental punishment per 100 facilities across states. It should be kept in mind that the punishment rates are inflated by several limitations in the data (e.g., they are calculated for three and five year periods).

Having summarized variability in known environmental offending and punishment across states, we now turn to assessing potential state-level correlates of environmental crime.

6.8 EPA Regional Variation in Environmental Crimes

Previously, we discussed two Models (1 and 2) that suggested regional variability in environmental crimes, and a possible organizational component to regional variability. This section examines that variability further, displaying minimum, maximum and mean values for CEVR and 3YNCR by EPA region. These results are shown in Tables 6.1 and 6.2.

As seen in Table 6.1, minimum variation in CEVR across EPA regions is fairly substantial. Region 5 contains the state with the lowest CEVR (0.74/100 facilities), which is less than one-half of the next lowest rate (region 2). More noteworthy, region 10 contains the largest minimum CEVR and the largest maximum CEVR. Whether these high minimums and maximums reflect more environmental offending or more diligent enforcement efforts is a question that requires further research. Also notable is that the next highest minimum and maximums co-occur in the same region, region 6. The lowest minimum and maximum CEVRs do not co-occur in the same region. The lowest CEVR (0.74/100 facilities) occurs in

Table 6.1 EPA regional variation in current violation rates per 100 facilities

EPA region	Current min	Current max	Current mean	Current SD	N states
1	3.41	14.09	8.522	4.693	6
2	3.42	5.10	4.26	1.184	2
3	2.40	8.35	4.971	2.736	5
4	1.97	9.80	5.655	2.483	8
5	0.74	13.41	6.330	4.386	6
6	6.07	21.45	11.295	6.431	5
7	2.10	12.52	7.540	4.504	4
8	4.47	14.78	8.512	3.725	6
9	3.08	13.48	6.121	4.961	4
10	12.95	29.26	21.414	7.611	4

Table 6.2 EPA regional variation in three year noncompliance rate (3YNCR) per 100 facilities

EPA region	3-year min	3-year max	3-year mean	3-year SD	N states
1	11.74	37.51	25.530	11.183	6
2	11.90	17.29	14.596	3.806	2
3	8.48	20.48	14.247	4.632	5
4	6.21	37.38	18.325	9.522	8
5	5.67	29.69	17.701	9.762	6
6	11.95	39.24	24.068	12.325	5
7	5.84	20.47	15.975	6.909	4
8	10.91	39.68	22.254	9.502	6
9	6.94	33.65	17.557	12.090	4
10	26.84	58.39	43.473	13.325	4

region 5 (Minnesota), and the lowest maximum CEVR (5.1), is found in Region 2 (New York).

Table 6.2 assesses variation in 3YNCR across US EPA regions. The data in this Table also indicates that the highest minimum and highest maximum rates are found in region 10. Consistent with Table 6.1 for CEVR, the lowest minimum 3YNCR rate is found in region 5. In contrast to Table 6.1 where the second highest maximum CEVR was found in region 6, in Table 6.2 the second largest maximum 3YNCR rate is found in region 8.

Tables 6.1 and 6.2 suggest some geographic overlap between these two measures of environmental crime. Indeed, the geographic distribution of CEVR and 3YNCR are highly correlated ($r = 0.897$, $p = 0.0000$). In short, the EPA region data indicates the potential existence of a geographic distribution of environmental crime. The next section examines some possible correlates of environmental crime across states derived from a variety of studies we cannot review in detail here (see, Lynch et al. 2017a, b).

6.9 Predictors of Environmental Crime and Punishment Rates Across States

This section summarizes a series of regression models employed to assess associations between state level characteristics and known environmental crimes across states. These analyses are divided into three parts that examine state: (1) structural characteristics; (2) economic characteristics; and (3) population characteristics. Findings from these regression analyses were then combined to detect the most persistent or strongest correlates.

1. State structural variables. Model 3 (not shown) assessed effects of state structural variables on environmental crime. State structural variables measure state geographic characteristics and some population measures hypothesized to enhance or diminish the likelihood of environmental crime. These variables were used to predict CEVR (Models 3A and 3B) or 3NRC (Model 3C and 3D). The variables primarily focused on opportunity, and included: (1) miles of rivers and streams; (2) miles of shoreline (lakes and ocean); (3) percent urban land area; (4) population density (population per acre); (5) percent of state that is grassland; (6) agricultural land; and (7) percent of state that is forested. Miles of river and streams were drawn from US EPA documents [2], and US Coastline data from the National Oceanic and Atmospheric Administration [3]. Waterways are subject to numerous environmental protection laws, and present opportunities for environmental crimes to occur. As a result, the rate of environmental offending across states could be impacted by waterway access.

Percent urban, forest, agricultural, and grass land area, were extracted from US Department of Agricultural data, and measure whether cross-state land use impacts the opportunity for environmental crime. Many polluting facilities (e.g. factories) are located in urban areas, and thus the percentage of urban land in a state may increase the rate of environmental crime. An alternative measure of development is population density. Since population density and percent urban area are highly correlated, their effects were assessed in separate regression models. Conversely, the percentage of land employed for agriculture, or preserved in forests and grassland is expected to be inversely related to environmental crimes generated by polluting facilities.

Four versions of Model 3 were estimated: (A) for CEVR with percent urban land, but not population density; (B) for CEVR with population density, but not percent urban land; (C) for 3NCR with percent urban land; and (D) for 3NCR with population density. All estimated models were quite inefficient, with adjusted R-square values between 2.4 and 5.4% and no independent variables were significant in any model. Thus, we rejected the assumption that these state structural variables have an impact on the distribution of known environmental offending across states.

2. *State Economic Characteristics.* A wide variety of indicators could be employed to measure state economic characteristics. Here, we employed: (1) state gross domestic product per capita (US Census Bureau); (2) mean state income (US Census Bureau); (3) BTU use per capita (US Energy Information Administration)

and (4) a measure of land within each state devoted to manufacturing and defense industry sector development (US Department of Agriculture). Theoretically, economic development has been linked to environmental pollution through research on the Environmental Kuznets Curve (EKC; Dinda 2004; Grossman and Krueger 1995; for a green critique see, Lynch 2016a). The EKC argument suggests that during early stages of development, increasing economic development causes an increase in pollution. At some point, however, additional economic development generates declining levels of pollution, perhaps as a result of rising incomes which generate increased public pressure for environmental protection. With respect to environmental crime, one could argue that the effect of development on crime should be the opposite of the effect on pollution—that is, if increased development enhances public expectations for environmental protection, then development should lead to enhanced environmental protection and an increasing rate of environmental offenses.

We tested these assumptions in Models 4A (CEVR) and Model 4B (3YNCR; not shown). Both Models fit the data poorly, with adjusted R-squares near zero, and no statistically significant effects.

In Models 5A (CEVR) and Model 5B (3YNCR; not shown), we assessed whether indicators of inequality might be related to environmental offending. There is a significant literature on environmental justice (Chakraborty 2012; Holifield et al. 2017), which posits that exposure to environmental pollution is affected by community class, race and ethnic characteristics (e.g., Carson et al. 1997; Pastor et al. 2004; for a green criminological review see Lynch et al. 2015). In addition, prior research indicates a relationship between the unequal distribution of power and environmental controls (Boyce 1994; Boyce et al. 1999). The variables included in Model 5A/B were state level Gini coefficient, poverty rate and percent Black population. Of these variables, percent non-Hispanic-Black was the only predictor that illustrated some potential effect (3YNCR, $p = 0.058$; CEVR, $p = 0.085$).

Model 6 assessed effects for five variables that have not been employed in prior studies: (1) The volume of coal, in tons, produced within each state, which can affect environmental violations related to water and air pollution; (2) the number of oil refineries within a state, since oil refineries generate water, air, and land pollution; (3) a count of the largest 100 coal-ash ponds across US states, since such sites can produce water pollution problems; (4) the volume of tons shipped by rail, since rail shipments are used to move commodities such as chemicals, oil and gasoline as well as toxic waste, and thus the volume of rail shipments may impact the opportunity for environmental offenses; and (5) the dollar value of average welfare payments in a state as an indicator of a state's commitment to the welfare of its citizens. We also included the percent non-Hispanic Black indicator identified in Model 5 in Model 6 analyses as a potentially important predictor of environmental crime's distribution.

The results from Model 6A (CEVR) and 6B (3NCR) produced several notable results. In Model 6A, percent non-Hispanic Black ($b = -0.271$; $p = 0.003$), average welfare payment ($b = -0.001$; $p = 0.007$), and number of oil refineries ($b = 0.564$;

p = 0.036) were statistically significant predictors (adjusted R-square = 0.222) of CEVR. In Model 6B, average welfare payment was again significant (b = −0.001; p = 0.012), while the effect of percent non-Hispanic Black was negative but marginal (p = 0.054), and the effect for oil refineries was insignificant.

With respect environmental justice issues, the negative effect for percent non-Hispanic Black indicates that states with larger Black populations have reduced environmental protection. Given findings in the environmental justice literature that African American communities are more proximate to environmental hazards, this result suggests that lower levels of discovering environmental crime adversely impact African American communities. Due to the level of aggregation in the current study, however, such a conclusion is only suggestive and requires further research (e.g., Lynch et al. 2004a, b), and such studies should also attend to findings indicating that at local levels, polluting facilities also engage in creating "recipes of risk" (Grant et al. 2010).

3. State Population Characteristics. Prior environmental studies indicate that state population characteristics such as education (Boyce 1994) and voter turnout (Boyce et al. 1999) are related to environmental protection and pollution exposure. Beyond such studies, there is little guidance for selecting other state population characteristics that might influence the volume of environmental crime. We measured education using the percent of college graduates, which should increase pressure for environmental regulations and potentially the rate of environmental offending through increased enforcement. We also included voter turnout, believed to increase environmental protection when voter turnout is high (Boyce 1994). To these more common measures, we added the Mercatus Center measure of state level "personal freedoms." We hypothesized that as the Mercatus score increased, signaling an increase in personal freedom and reduced state control, the volume of environmental crime would decline. The Mercatus freedom index uses three constructs, each composed of several variables: (1) fiscal policy freedoms (comprised of tax burden, government employment, government spending, government debt and fiscal decentralization); (2) regulatory policy freedoms (freedom from tort abuse, property rights protection, health insurance freedom, labor market freedom, regulatory freedom, and cable and telecom freedom); and (3) indicators of personal freedom (victimless crime freedom, gun control freedom, tobacco freedom, alcohol freedom, marriage freedom, marijuana and salvia freedom, gambling freedom, educational policy, civil liberties, travel freedom, assets forfeiture freedom and campaign finance reform).

These effects of the variables described above were assessed in Models 7A (CEVR) and 7B (3NCR). In these models we retained percent Black due to effects noted in prior models.

In Models 7A and 7B, only percent Black showed any evidence of an effect. In 7A (CEVR) the effect of percent non-Hispanic Black was negative (p = 0.027), while in 7B, its effect, still negative, were marginal (p = 0.063). However, the predictive power (adjusted R-square) of these models was quite low (13% for 7A and 6% for 7B), indicating that the predictors are not strongly related to the outcomes. In sum, the models measuring state population characteristics rejected most of the associations examined.

4. Reassessment of Effects Controlling for EPA Regions. Earlier results indicated EPA region effects. Models 8 (A and B) and 9 (A and B) assessed this relationship further controlling for environmental punishment: Model 8A and 9A included ER1, and Model 8B and 9B, ER2. In addition, we retained significant variables (percent non-Hispanic Black, welfare, and oil refinery) from the regressions estimated above. Controlling for EPA region removed the effect of percent non-Hispanic Black and number of oil refineries across all four models (see Table 6.3 for results). With respect to the enforcement rate measures, only ER2 showed an effect in one

Table 6.3 Current (Model 8A and B) and 3-year environmental violation (Model 9A and B) OLS models[a]

Variable	Model 8A	Model 8B	Model 9A	Model 9B
Percent black	−0.087(0.098) [0.381]	−0.102(0.098) [0.304)	0.003(0.220) [0.989]	−0.040(0.215) [0.853]
Welfare	−0.001(0.001) [0.002]	−0.001(0.001) [0.033]	−0.001(0.000) [0.002]	−0.001[0.000) [0.071]
Oil refineries	0.110(0.114) [0.448]	0.176(0.148) [0.242]	−0.210(0.323) [0.521]	−0.009[0.325) [0.977]
EPA 1	−9.401(2.776) [0.002]	−9.137(2.783) [0.002]	−11.963(6.240) [0.063]	−11.013(6.121) [0.080]
EPA 2	−12.331(3.819) [0.003]	−11.666(3.843) [0.004]	−20.570(8.585) [0.022]	−18.456(8.452) [0.036]
EPA 3	−12.251(3.066) [0.000]	−13.408(3.130) [0.000]	−27.505(6.891) [0.000]	−24.746(6.884) [0.001]
EPA 4	−16.197(3.348) [0.000]	−13.256(3.585) [0.001]	−30.927(7.526) [0.000]	−22.402(7.885) [0.007]
EPA 5	−14.132(2.742) [0.000)	−14.071(2.739) [0.000]	−24.980(6.163) [0.000]	−24.477(6.024) [0.000]
EPA 6	−11.822(3.102) [0.001)	−9.832(3.163) [0.004]	−22.134(6.972) [0.003]	−16.294(6.956) [0.025]
EPA 7	−13.666(2.948) [0.000]	−13.518(2.954) [0.000]	−28.282(6.627) [0.000]	−27.482(6.496) [0.000]
EPA 8	−12.673(2.623) [0.000]	−12.773(2.610) [0.000]	−20.202(5.987) [0.002)	−20.276(5.741) [0.001]
EPA 9	−12.392(2.989) [0.000]	−12.274(2.982) [0.000]	−18.972(6.719) [0.008]	−18.582(6.558) [0.007]
E-Rate1	0.336(0.220) [0.135]	–	0.874(0.494) [0.086]	–
E-Rate2	–	−6.516(4.166) [0.122]	–	−20.359(9.053) [0.031]
Constant	29.360(3.516) [0.000]	28.741(3.588) [0.000]	60.792(7.903) [0.000]	58.390(7.892) [0.000]
Adj. R-square	0.543	0.545	0.406	0.434

[a]b, (S.E.) [p] values

model (9B). Welfare dollars per welfare recipient is significant in all models except 9B, and is negatively related to the rate of environmental crimes known. These models suggest that controlling for punishment (which was insignificant), EPA region is the most important predictor of environmental crime, and that welfare expenditures generally has an effect. States that spend more on welfare per recipient have a lower rate of known environmental crimes, which may indicate that states with a greater concern for social welfare have lower rates of environmental offending.

The above models were also re-estimated using log-transformed variables (not shown) to determine if the results may be an artifact of the distribution of the variables and their use in OLS. The transformed models were quite similar to the non-transformed results. The notable differences relate to the effect of two EPA Regions, 1 and 2. In the logged models, Regions 1 and 2, which together make up the northeastern states, are now not statistically different from the effect of Region 10. When the logged model are employed to estimate the three-year violation rate outcome, only EPA Region 2 is statistically non-different than Region 10.

5. Additional Regression Analysis. Above, few variables predicted variations in environmental violations across states. We ran numerous additional models (not shown) attempting to predict cross state variations in CEVR and 3YNCR, which were largely unsuccessful. Two additional variables, however—the ratio of the non-Hispanic Black to non-Hispanic White population (W/B), and percent land in each state owned by the federal government (FedLand)—showed evidence of an effect controlling for EPA Regions and average welfare expenditures. In these models, we employed the W/B ratio as an alternative measure of environmental justice to examine the geographic relationship between race and environmental hazards.

Model 10A (CEVR) and 10B (3YNCR) included controls for EPA Region and welfare. In Model 10A (Adj. R-square = 0.610), both W/B ratio ($b = 0.001$; $p = 0.42$) and FedLand ($b = -0.125$; $p = 0.02$) were statistically related to the CEVR. For W/B, the larger the ratio of Whites to Blacks (i.e., more whites), the higher the CEVR. This finding may be an indicator of a form of environmental injustice where states with more predominately white populations pay greater attention to environmental violations. The negative relationship between FedLand and the CEVR may indicate less opportunity for environmental violations by facilities in states where a larger percentage of land is owned by the federal government and preserved in federal parks.

In Model 10B (3YNCR), controlling for EPA region and welfare, FedLand was not significant, while W/B ratio was ($b = 0.002$; S. E. = 0.001; $p = 0.009$). Here, as in Model 10A, the positive effect of W/B may indicate an environmental justice effect where states with a higher concentration of White populations are more likely to discover environmental violations at facilities.

Log-transformed models (not shown) displayed similar results. Those models, however, indicated some interaction between welfare and the white/black population ratio. When these variables are both entered into the regression, the effect of welfare is significant, but the white/black ratio is not. When welfare is removed, the white/black ratio is significant. This may indicate a long-known race-class-income interaction. These interactions are difficult to disentangle. While one can argue this can be done statistically, the concern is that race-class-income interactions are not simply mathematical problems, but rather are social process interactions that may escape adequate empirical modeling efforts.

6.10 Discussion

The current study provided an initial, wide-ranging examination of variations in environmental crimes across US states to examine the geography of environmental crime and its correlates. The data were limited to violations by permitted facilities (Clean Air Act, Clean Water Act, and Resource Conservation and Recovery facilities) and facilities in each state that filed Toxic Release Inventory reports.

First, we found widespread variability in the number and rate of current environmental offenses, three year noncompliance and formal enforcement. The number of current environmental violations varied by a factor of 56 between the low and high count states, and as a rate by more than 3850% across states; three year noncompliance offenses varied from 298 to 9026, and as a rate by more than 930%; the number of enforcement actions over five years varied from 14 to 3467 across states, with a low of 0.76 actions per 100 violators to a high of 19.65 per 100. The extent of variation noted in environmental offending is much more widespread than the variation in street crime rates across states, and suggests that sensitivity to controlling and enforcing environmental laws is much more volatile than for street crime.

Second, we found that measures of environmental crime rates across states (CEVR and 3YNCR) were unrelated to rates of street crime offending, suggesting either that the causes of environmental and street crime offending or the enforcement of environmental and street crime laws (or both) require different kinds of explanations.

Third, we noted that environmental crime is likely more widespread than street crime, especially with respect to its victimization effects (i.e., has more victims, and the victims span across groups including human and nonhuman beings), prior studies have not measured this association due to a failure to employ available geographic data. In short, prior studies have not compared the concentration of street and environmental crime rates across state. Doing so, we found that on average across states, environmental crime rates were three times higher or more concentrated than street crime rates. Fourth, in addition we also found that variations in environmental crime across states consisted of regional variability linked to EPA regions.

Fifth, using various regression analyses that assessed the effects of 36 potential correlates of environmental offending for both CEVR and 3NCR, we found few correlates of green crimes. Those correlates included EPA region, the White/Black

Table 6.4 Summary results, 36 predictors of current environmental violation (CREV) and 3-year noncompliance (3YNCR) rates across states; (SS = statistically significant, positive [+] or negative [−]; NS = not significant)

	CREV	3YNCR	Comments
UCR violent crime rate	NS	SS ($p = 0.018$)	Controlling for EPA regions
UCR property crime rate	NS	NS	
EPA regions[a]	ALL	ALL	
Ave. welfare payment	SS−	SS−	Controlling for EPA Regions
Rivers/stream miles	NS	NS	
Lake/ocean miles	NS	NS	
%Urban	NS	NS	
Pop. density	NS	NS	
Grassland	NS	NS	
Agricultural land	NS	NS	
Forest area	NS	NS	
State GDP	NS	NS	
Mean income	NS	NS	
BTU/capita	NS	NS	
Man./defense industries	NS	NS	
GINI	NS	NS	
%Black	NS	NS	
Coal tons	NS	NS	
N oil refineries	NS	NS	
Coal ash ponds	NS	NS	
Rail tons shipped	NS	NS	
State freedom index	NS	NS	
% BS degrees	NS	NS	
E-Rate1	NS	NS	
E-Rate2	NS	NS	
W/B	S+	S+	
FedLand	S−	NS	

[a]Compared to the omitted category, region 10, all other regions have a negative, significant effect as expected

ratio, and state welfare payments (see Table 6.4 for summary of effects across all Models).

The most consistent environmental offense correlate was EPA Region, indicating an organizational/regional component to the distribution of environmental offenses. This finding suggests that future research examine differences in the focus of EPA regions as one possible explanation for variations in environmental crime rates across states. Data for such studies should draw on US EPA files under the "State Review Framework for Compliance and Enforcement Performance" (the SRF program; accessed December 6th, 2015; http://www.epa.gov/compliance/state-review-framework-compliance-and-enforcement-performance), which specifically examines US EPA and state enforcement of the CWA, CAA and RCRA Acts. The EPA uses these data "to ensure fair and consistent enforcement and compliance programs across states." Findings from the present study related to variations in CEVR and 3YNCR across states related to EPA regions suggests that perhaps EPA has yet to accomplish this goal.

Besides significant regional variation, other notable effects were found for the ratio of the White to Black population (W/B), and average welfare payments. The W/B results suggest that states with higher concentrations of White populations discover more environmental violations at facilities, which may be interpreted as a form of environmental injustice and enhanced efforts to protect areas where White populations are concentrated from environmental crime. This result is also, we suggest, inconsistent with the EPA's claims about fairness and equity in environmental enforcement drawn from its SRF webpage, but is consistent with lower level aggregation studies of environmental justice.

The other persistent effect we found was for average welfare payments. As noted, as average welfare payments increased, the rate of environmental offending, whether measured as CEVR or 3YNCR, declined controlling for other variables. This outcome may suggest that states with greater concern for the poor, do a better job of discovering environmental violations. How this finding and the W/B finding are integrated with respect to the analysis of environmental justice is an interesting question requiring further research. It is possible that state racial composition and poverty intersect or interact, and that the independent effects for welfare and W/B indicate a much more complex relationship than we can disentangle here (e.g., effects of welfare and poverty rates by race and ethnicity across states in relations to environmental crime rates).

While we have focused on the geography and correlates of environmental crime across states, few studies address this issue *within* states (Hammett and Epstein 1993; Pollock and Vittas 1995; Uhlmann 2014), and little is known about the kinds of environmental crimes that are discovered or prosecuted, or the volume and types of environmental crimes different states experience. Thus, there are numerous studies on environmental crime that need to be undertaken before we know about these offenses. Those studies are necessary because they change what is known about crime, since the vast majority of what is claimed to be known about crime come only from the study of street crime.

The nature of this research was preliminary. As a result, here we were less concerned with some technical and methodological specification issues, and more interested in discovering if there was potential evidence of state-level environmental crime patterns that could be explored in greater depth in future research. Nevertheless, there are limitations to our research that should be mentioned.

As noted, our measure of environmental crime was limited to pollution offenses, leaving out a large volume of environmental offenses. Many of those offenses involve violations against wildlife, domestic/companion animals, farm animals and laboratory animals. Crimes against wildlife can include a range of crimes (e.g., illegal hunting, fishing, trapping; illegal trade/possession of game animals; wildlife trafficking; etc.,). There are also a large number of harms against farm and laboratory animals. Added together, these latter crimes far exceed those related to pollution, and those crimes may have a completely different distribution than pollution-related green crimes (Crow et al. 2013; Lynch and Genco 2018; Pires and Clarke 2011, 2012; Petrossian and Clarke 2013; Stretesky et al. 2018).

In addition to the above, other ways of measuring the dependent variable could clearly affect the outcome. The green crimes in our study were an aggregation of Clean Air Act, Clean Water Act, Resource Conservation Recovery Act, and Toxic Release Inventory violations. It is possible that each individual type of offense has its own unique ecological distribution across states, different predictors, and relationship to street crime. In another unpublished work, we have been examining related models for emissions from Publicly Owned Treatment Works (POTWs) that treat and release treated water (see also, Lynch et al. 2017a, b). Like the violations here, the ecological distribution of POTW pollution is difficult to predict.

The sample size for the data was impacted by using states. One could increase the sample by collecting the data we employed over time as well. That is possible using other EPA data sources beyond those used here. In addition, we began with states given that little is known about the distribution of green crimes, and cross state analysis is a useful level of aggregation to begin building information about the distribution of green crimes. Clearly, however, examining the geography of green crimes can also be performed at lower levels of analysis within and across states using data from cities, or counties, census tracts, zip codes or block groups. Lower level analysis would tell a much different story than the one written here across states. Indeed, within cities, it has already been argued that one would expect street crime and environmental crime to overlap in ways that reflect the political economic organization of cities and urban power structures as part of the urban geography or advantage and disadvantage (Lynch 2016b). That argument can also be connected to related literature in environmental justice, which is quite large, and to arguments and empirical results contained in the green criminological literature (Lynch et al. 2015; Stretesky and Lynch 1998, 1999, 2002, 2011). There are numerous neighborhood class, race, ethnicity, poverty, etc., conditions that could be examined at lower levels of analysis. Part of the point here, however, is that these analyses have not been done within the green criminological literature, leaving many research questions open for exploration.

Our cross state results were likely also impacted by choices we made about variable transformations. In preliminary works, our preference is to examine the data using as few transformations as possible. While sometimes doing so violates assumptions of OLS, OLS analysis tends to be robust enough to discover relevant predictor despite violations of assumptions. Clearly, however, future analysis should take those violations more seriously to research more definitive conclusions than those produced here as part of this preliminary assessment. In the current study, one of the key factors we believed would impact the distribution of environmental crimes across states was the differential implementation of policies and procedures, and resource distributions across US EPA regions. Our data indeed indicated significant EPA region effects. Knowing those effects exist would likely change how future studies model cross state environmental crimes, which involve procedures we did not take up here.

In closing, we note that one can imagine a whole range of studies that replicate more traditional criminological studies of the correlates of crime across geographic areas that can be applied to environmental crimes. Moreover, there are specific or different kinds of green crimes, and each of these may have their own unique geographic distribution. For example, toxic environmental crimes committed by corporations will vary geographically along with characteristics of the industries in which those corporations are embedded. Thus, some types of green corporate crimes will have geographic distributions associated with characteristics of urban landscapes (e.g., manufacturing, chemical production), while others (e.g., mining), will have rural geographic patterns. The geography of wildlife crimes may be more heavily concentrated in rural areas, although for some crimes, perhaps fishing violations (which geographically also require considering the geography of water), fish-violation hotspots might emerge in large urban centers with waterway access. And, we would argue, before criminologists can say they "know" about crime these kinds of studies need to be undertaken and integrated into the criminological literature. It is only after such additional analysis and integration that the biases constructed, contained within and communicated by criminology can be erased (Lynch 2015).

Endnotes

1. Because the EPA data uses a rolling indicator, these rankings and the distribution noted here is likely to change somewhat over time.
2. http://water.epa.gov/lawsregs/guidance/cwa/305b/upload/2000_06_28_305b_98report_appenda.pdf.
3. US Department of Commerce, National Oceanic and Atmospheric Administration. (1975). The Coastline of the United States. Washington, DC: USGPO. http://www.nauticalcharts.noaa.gov/hsd/docs/CSE_library_Coastline_of_the_US_1975.pdf.

Appendix

Number of Current Environmental Violation (Current N, CEV), Rate of Current Violations Per 100 Facilities (Current Rate, CEVR), Three Year Number of Noncompliance Case (3-Year N, 3NC), Rate of Three Year Noncompliance per 100 Facilities (3-Year Rate, 3NCR), Number of Formal Enforcement Actions Last 5 Years (Enforcement N), Formal Enforcement Rate per 100 Facilities (Enforcement Rate1, ER1), and Ratio Enforcement Rate to 3 Year Noncompliance Rate (Enforcement Rate2, ER2) from US EPA Environmental Compliance History Online. (Accessed December 8, 2015)

State	Current N (CEV)	Current rate (CEVR)	3-year N (3NC)	3-year rate (3NCR)	Enforcement N	Enforcement Rate1 (ER1)	Enforcement Rate2 (ER2)
Alabama	831	4.49	2472	13.36	538	2.91	0.218
Alaska	1313	17.23	2045	26.84	174	2.28	0.085
Arizona	658	13.48	1643	33.65	143	2.93	0.087
Arkansas	1002	13.74	2861	39.24	599	8.22	0.209
California	1852	3.08	4169	6.94	2781	4.63	0.667
Colorado	1285	4.47	3138	10.91	644	2.24	0.205
Connecticut	899	11.79	1866	24.46	442	5.79	0.237
Delaware	136	7.47	372	20.43	81	4.45	0.218
Florida	1130	1.97	3564	6.21	1091	1.90	0.306
Georgia	749	6.37	2450	20.83	606	5.15	0.247
Hawaii	98	3.20	298	9.73	97	3.17	0.326
Idaho	716	26.22	1320	48.33	144	5.27	0.109
Illinois	2389	5.12	4288	9.19	1120	2.40	0.261
Indiana	1035	7.89	3896	29.69	932	7.10	0.239
Iowa	1068	9.56	2265	20.27	372	3.33	0.164
Kansas	498	2.10	1382	5.84	354	1.50	0.256
Kentucky	1913	9.80	4001	20.51	552	2.83	0.138
Louisiana	2608	6.63	4702	11.95	2130	5.41	0.453
Maine	564	14.09	1502	37.51	154	3.85	0.103
Maryland	601	2.40	2120	8.48	579	2.31	0.273
Massachusetts	596	3.83	1974	12.67	1418	9.10	0.718
Michigan	928	3.26	4450	15.65	449	1.58	0.101
Minnesota	175	0.74	1346	5.67	468	1.97	0.348
Mississippi	396	6.23	2375	37.38	306	4.82	0.129
Missouri	3690	12.52	6032	20.47	478	1.62	0.079
Montana	775	14.78	2080	39.68	231	4.41	0.111
Nebraska	423	5.98	1226	17.33	229	3.24	0.187
Nevada	112	4.72	472	19.90	63	2.66	0.133
New Hampshire	237	5.86	1320	32.62	148	3.66	0.112
New Jersey	691	3.42	2403	11.90	1045	5.18	0.435
New Mexico	481	6.07	1248	15.76	372	4.70	0.298
New York	2607	5.10	8840	17.29	2276	4.45	0.257
North Carolina	1390	7.88	3709	21.02	3467	19.65	0.935
North Dakota	124	6.70	340	18.38	14	0.76	0.041
Ohio	2642	7.57	6286	18.00	571	1.64	0.091
Oklahoma	1129	8.58	2380	18.10	967	7.35	0.406
Oregon	609	12.95	1897	40.33	235	5.00	0.124
Pennsylvania	1526	3.60	6263	14.78	1554	3.67	0.248
Rhode Island	153	3.41	526	11.74	175	3.90	0.333
South Carolina	361	3.46	968	9.28	396	3.80	0.409
South Dakota	219	9.20	521	21.88	67	2.81	0.129

(continued)

(continued)

State	Current N (CEV)	Current rate (CEVR)	3-year N (3NC)	3-year rate (3NCR)	Enforcement N	Enforcement Rate1 (ER1)	Enforcement Rate2 (ER2)
Tennessee	486	5.04	1738	18.02	502	5.21	0.289
Texas	5485	21.45	9026	35.29	1812	7.08	0.201
Utah	410	10.12	908	22.40	142	3.50	0.156
Vermont	408	12.16	1146	34.17	28	0.83	0.024
Virginia	518	3.03	1912	11.17	386	2.26	0.202
Washington	2518	29.26	5025	58.39	545	6.33	0.108
West Virginia	861	8.35	1688	16.38	646	6.27	0.383
Wisconsin	1981	13.41	4173	28.24	201	1.36	0.048
Wyoming	379	5.80	1324	20.27	430	6.58	0.325
State MEAN	**1071**	**8.31**	**2679**	**21.37**	**663.61**	**4.26**	**0.243**
State LOW	**98**	**0.74**	**298**	**5.67**	**14**	**0.76**	**0.02**
State HIGH	**5485**	**29.26**	**9026**	**58.39**	**3467**	**19.65**	**0.93**

References

Allan, E. A., & Steffensmeier, D. J. (1989). Youth, underemployment, and property crime: Differential effects of job availability and job quality on juvenile and young adult arrest rates. *American Sociological Review, 54*(1), 107–123.

Beirne, P. (1999). For a nonspeciesist criminology: Animal abuse as an object of study. *Criminology, 37*(1), 117–148.

Boyce, J. K. (1994). Inequality as a cause of environmental degradation. *Ecological Economics, 11*(3), 169–178.

Boyce, J. K., Klemer, A. R., Templet, P. H., & Willis, C. E. (1999). Power distribution, the environment, and public health: A state-level analysis. *Ecological Economics, 29*(1), 127–140.

Brisman, A., & South, N. (2013). A green-cultural criminology: An exploratory outline. *Crime, Media, Culture, 9*(2), 115–135.

Carson, R. T., Jeon, Y., & McCubbin, D. R. (1997). The relationship between air pollution emissions and income: US data. *Environment and Development Economics, 2*(4), 433–450.

Chakraborty, J. (2012). Cancer risks from exposure to hazardous air pollutants: Spatial and social inequalities in Tampa Bay, Florida. *International Journal of Environmental Health Research, 22*(2), 165–183.

Chamlin, M. B., and Cochran, J. K. (1995). Assessing messner and Rosenfeld's institutional anomie theory: A partial test. *Criminology 33*(3): 411–429.

Chamlin, M. B., & Cochran, J. K. (1997). Social altruism and crime. *Criminology, 35*(2), 203–226.

Chintrakarn, P., & Herzer, D. (2012). More inequality, more crime? A panel cointegration analysis for the United States. *Economics Letters, 116*(3), 389–391.

Cohen, M. A. (1992). Environmental crime and punishment: Legal/economic theory and empirical evidence on enforcement of federal environmental statutes. *Journal of Criminal Law and Criminology 82*(4): 1054–1108.

Crow, M., Shelley, T. O. C., & Stretesky, P. B. (2013). Camouflage-collar crime: An examination of wildlife crime and characteristics of offenders in Florida. *Deviant Behavior, 34*(8), 635–652.

Dinda, S. (2004). Environmental Kuznets curve hypothesis: A survey. *Ecological Economics, 49,* 431–455.

Goyes, D. R., & South, N. (2015). Land-grabs, biopiracy and the inversion of justice in Colombia. *British Journal of Criminology 56*(3): 558–577.

Grant, D., Trautner, M. N., Downey, L., & Thiebaud, L. (2010). Bringing the polluters back in: Environmental inequality and the organization of chemical production. *American Sociological Review 75*(4): 479–504.

Grossman, G. M., & Krueger, A. B. (1995). Economic growth and the environment. *Quarterly Journal of Economics, 60,* 353–377.

Hammett, T. M., & Epstein, J. (1993). *Local prosecution of environmental crime*. United States Department of Justice, Office of Justice Programs. Washington, DC: National Institute of Justice.

Holifield, R., Chakraborty, J., & Walker, G. (Eds.). (2017). *The Routledge handbook of environmental justice*. London: Routledge.

Kawachi, I., Kennedy, B. P., & Wilkinson, R. G. (1999). Crime: Social disorganization and relative deprivation. *Social Science and Medicine, 48*(6), 719–731.

Land, K. C., McCall, P. L., & Cohen, L. E. (1990). Structural covariates of homicide rates: Are there any invariances across time and social space? *American Journal of Sociology, 95*(4), 922–963.

Lynch, M. J. (1990). The greening of criminology: A perspective for the 1990s. *The Critical Criminologist 2*(3):3–4, 11–12.

Lynch, M. J. (2015). The classless state of criminology and why criminology without class is rather meaningless. *Crime, Law and Social Change, 63*(1), 65–90.

Lynch, M. J. (2016a). A Marxian interpretation of the environmental Kuznets curve: Global capitalism and the rise, fall (and rise) of pollution. *Capitalism, Nature, Socialism, 27*(4), 77–95.

Lynch, M. J. (2016b). The ecological distribution of community advantage and disadvantage: Power structures, political economy, communities, and green-state crime and justice. *Critical Criminology, 24*(2), 247–262.

Lynch, M. J. (2017). The sentencing/punishment of federal environmental criminal offenses, 2000–2013. *Deviant Behavior, 38*(9), 991–1008.

Lynch, M. J., & Genco, L. (2018). Animal Abuse registries: Expanded interest in animal protection mimics other criminal justice policies, but should green criminologists hop on the band-wagon? *Contemporary Justice Review, 21*(4), 351–370.

Lynch, M. J., & Pires, S. F. (2019). Quantitative studies in green and conservation criminology. In M. J. Lynch & S. F. Pires (Eds.), *Quantitative studies in green and conservation criminology: The measurement of environmental harm and crime*. New York: Routledge.

Lynch, M. J., & Stretesky, P. B. (2001). Toxic crimes: Examining corporate victimization of the general public employing medical and epidemiological evidence. *Critical Criminology, 10*(3), 153–172.

Lynch, M. J., & Stretesky, P. B. (2013). The distribution of water-monitoring organizations across states: Implications for community policing. *Policing: An International Journal of Police Strategies and Management 36*(1): 6–26.

Lynch, M. J., Stretesky, P. B., & Burns, R. G. (2004a). Determinants of environmental law violation fines against oil refineries: Race, ethnicity, income and aggregation effects. *Society and Natural Resources, 17*(4), 333–347.

Lynch, M. J., Stretesky, P. B., & Burns, R. G. (2004b). Slippery business: Race, class and legal determinants of penalties against petroleum refineries. *Journal of Black Studies, 34*(3), 421–440.

Lynch, M. J., Long, M. A., Barrett, K. L., & Stretesky, P. B. (2013). Is it a crime to produce ecological disorganization? why green criminology and political economy matter in the analysis of global ecological harms. *British Journal of Criminology, 53*(6), 997–1016.

Lynch, M. J., Stretesky, P. B., & Long, M. A. (2015). Environmental justice: A criminological perspective. *Environmental Research Letters, 10*(8), 085008.

Lynch, M. J., Barrett, K. L., Stretesky, P. B., & Long, M. A. (2016). The weak probability of punishment for environmental offenses and deterrence of environmental offenders: A discussion based on US EPA criminal cases, 1983–2013. *Deviant Behavior, 37*(10), 1095–1109.
Lynch, M. J., Barrett, K. L., Stretesky, P. B., & Long, M. A. (2017a). The neglect of quantitative research in green criminology and its consequences. *Critical Criminology, 25*(2), 183–198.
Lynch, M. J., Stretesky, P. B., & Long, M. A. (2017b). The state and green crimes related to water pollution and ecological additions: Water pollution from publicly owned water treatment (POTW) facilities across US states, a green criminological analysis. *Palgrave Communications* (open access). https://www.nature.com/articles/palcomms201770.
McCleary, R., Nienstedt, B. C., & Erven, J. M. (1982). Uniform crime reports as organizational outcomes: Three time series experiments. *Social Problems, 29*(4), 361–372.
McMurry, R. I., & Ramsey, S. D. (1986). Environmental crime: The use of criminal sanctions in enforcing environmental laws. *Loyola of Los Angeles Law Review, 19,* 1133–1170.
O'Hear, M. M. (2004). Sentencing the green-collar offender: Punishment, culpability, and environmental crime. *Journal of Criminal Law and Criminology, 95*(1), 133–276.
Pastor, M., Sadd, J. L., & Morello-Frosch, R. (2004). Waiting to inhale: The demographics of Toxic air release facilities in 21st-century California. *Social Science Quarterly, 85*(2), 420–440.
Petrossian, G. A., & Clarke, R. V. (2013). Explaining and controlling illegal commercial fishing an application of the CRAVED theft model. *British Journal of Criminology, 54*(1), 73–90.
Petrossian, G., Weis, J. S., & Pires, S. F. (2015). Factors affecting crab and lobster species subject to IUU fishing. *Ocean and Coastal Management, 106,* 29–34.
Pires, S. F., & Clarke, R. V. (2011). Sequential foraging, itinerant fences and parrot poaching in Bolivia. *British Journal of Criminology, 51*(2), 314–335.
Pires, S. F., & Clarke, R. V. (2012). Are parrots CRAVED? An analysis of parrot poaching in Mexico. *Journal of Research in Crime and Delinquency, 49*(1), 122–146.
Pollock, P. H., & Vittas, M. E. (1995). Who bearsthe burden of environmental pollution? Race, ethnicity, and environmental equity in Florida. *Social Science Quarterly, 76*(2), 294–210.
Quinney, R. (1966). Structural characteristics, population areas, and crime rates in the United States. *The Journal of Criminal Law, Criminology, and Police Science, 57*(1), 45–52.
Raphael, S., & Winter-Ebmer, R. (2001). Identifying the effect of unemployment on crime. *Journal of Law and Economics, 44*(1), 259–283.
Reiman, J. (1979). *The rich get richer and the poor get prison.* NY: Wiley.
Rosenfeld, R., Wallman, J., & Fornango, R. (2005). The contribution of ex-prisoners to crime rates. In J. Travis & C. Vishers (Eds.), *Prisoner reentry and crime in America* (pp. 80–104). NY: Cambridge University Press.
Stretesky, P. B., & Lynch, M. J. (1998). Corporate environmental violence and racism. *Crime, Law and Social Change, 30*(2), 163–184.
Stretesky, P. B., & Lynch, M. J. (1999). Environmental justice and the prediction of distance to accidental chemical releases in Hillsborough county Florida. *Social Science Quarterly, 80*(4), 830–846.
Stretesky, P. B., & Lynch, M. J. (2002). Environmental hazards and school segregation in Hillsborough, 1987–1999. *The Sociological Quarterly, 43*(4), 553–573.
Stretesky, P. B., & Lynch, M. J. (2009). Does self-policing reduce chemical emissions? A further test of the EPA self audit policy. *Social Science Research, 38*(1), 239–250.
Stretesky, P. B., & Lynch, M. J. (2011). Coal strip mining, mountain top removal and the distribution of environmental violations across the United States, 2002–2008. *Landscape Research, 36*(2), 209–230.
Stretesky, P. B., Long, M. A., & Lynch, M. J. (2013). *The treadmill of crime: Political economy and green criminology.* Abingdon, UK: Routledge.

Stretesky, P. B., McKie, R., Long, M. A., Lynch, M. J., & Barrett, K. L. (2018). Where have all the falcons gone? saker exports in a global economy. *Global Ecology and Conservation*. (Open access). *13*, e00372.

van Solinge, T. B. (2010). Deforestation crimes and conflicts in the Amazon. *Critical Criminology, 18*(4), 263–277.

Walters, R. (2007). Food crime, regulation and the biotech harvest. *European Journal of Criminology, 4*(2), 217–235.

Uhlmann, D. M. (2014). Prosecutorial discretion and environmental crime. *Harvard Environmental Law Review, 38*, 159–187.

Part III
Geography of Disorder

Chapter 7
Fear of Crime, Disorder, and Quality of Life

Michael Chataway and Alexandra Bourke

Fear of crime has been the focus of scientific investigation for over fifty years, with a number of potential correlates of crime fear identified during this time. The growing scholarship on fear of crime has suggested that feelings of worry or concern about crime and disorder may have a negative impact on quality of life and psychological wellbeing. In particular, research has suggested that fear of crime may contribute to active avoidance and withdrawal from people, situations and particular places, decreased life satisfaction, poor objective and subjective ratings of physical health, as well as increased hypervigilance and precautionary behaviour (Adams and Serpe 2000; Hanslmaier 2013; Stafford et al. 2007). In terms of societal consequences, high levels of fear of crime and visible disorder in neighbourhoods may erode social cohesion and contribute to a general mistrust of those responsible for "fighting" crime, such as law enforcement (Taylor et al. 1985). It is for these reasons, that reducing fear of crime has now become a government priority in most countries. This is further culminated by research evidencing that despite crime declining in most Western societies, fear of crime has remained relatively stable or increased over the past 30 years (Walker et al. 2006).

The primary purpose of this chapter is to provide a summary of some of the key developments in fear of crime research over the past few decades and how fear of crime may be related to perceptions of neighbourhood disorder. This chapter will begin by examining some of the different ways that fear of crime has been defined and operationalised, before proposing a new and useful working definition that considers fear of crime as a social-psychological process. This will be followed by a discussion of the common methods used to measure fear of crime and perceptions

M. Chataway (✉)
Queensland University of Technology, Brisbane, Australia
e-mail: michael.chataway@qut.edu.au

A. Bourke
Griffith University, Brisbane, Australia
e-mail: alexandra.bourke@griffithuni.edu.au

K. M. Lersch and J. Chakraborty (eds.), *Geographies of Behavioural Health, Crime, and Disorder*, GeoJournal Library 126,
https://doi.org/10.1007/978-3-030-33467-3_7

of disorder in neighbourhoods and public spaces. The second half of this chapter will describe the various correlates related to fear of crime, including individual-level variables such as gender and age; neighbourhood-level characteristics (such as disorder, socioeconomic status, and social disorganisation), and social characteristics (such as social capital, and informal social control). Moreover, we will discuss how these common predictors of fear of crime could be better converged into models. This chapter will conclude by discussing some new developments in the study of fear of crime, disorder, and quality of life, along with proposing recommendations for future research in these areas.

7.1 Defining and Operationalising Fear of Crime

Currently, no definitive meaning of fear of crime exists within the established literature. One of the earliest definitions of fear of crime is provided by Garofalo (1981), who asserts that "fear can be characterised by a sense of danger and anxiety produced by the threat of physical harm" (p. 840). Garofalo argues that to constitute fear of crime, a person's fear must be elicited by environmental cues that relate to some aspect of crime. From this definition one can assume that fear of crime is an affective (emotional) state associated with an anticipation of a looming threat in one's environment. Later definitions echo this early operationalisation of fear of crime by Garofalo, with Ferraro (1995) defining fear of crime as an "emotional response of dread or anxiety to crime or symbols that a person associates with crime" (p. 8).

Rather than focusing on specific emotional elements of fear of crime (i.e., anxiety or dread), some scholars have taken a much broader approach to its operationalisation. For example, Skogan (1976) defined fear of crime as a "diffuse psychological construct affected by a number of aspects of urban life" (p. 14). Skogan's definition captures the subjective social meanings behind fear of crime. That is, fear of crime may not be specifically about the 'experience' of crime, but may also encompass more perfuse concerns about oneself, society and social life—and may be construed through personal experiences (Hollway and Jefferson 1997; Lee 2008; Jackson 2004).

Warr (2000) argues that much of the problems associated with defining fear of crime stem from a failure to distinguish between three concepts: perception, emotion, and cognition. Moreover, for Warr, fear is not a perception of the environment, but rather a reaction to something within the environment. Warr argues that although fear may result from cognitive processing of perceptual information, fear is not in itself a belief, attitude, or evaluation. Instead, he argues that fear is an emotion, a feeling of anxiety that is caused by the anticipation of imminent danger. Fear of crime is no different from other forms of fear, such as fear of spiders, fear of tightly confined spaces, or fear of heights. Individual's "fears" are only differentiated by the object or stimulus that causes a fearful response (e.g., a spider, a tight space, a type of crime).

In so far, fear of crime has tended to be defined in affective terms, with most early theoretical pieces focusing on feelings of anxiety and dread in response to crime and disorder (Garofalo 1981; Ferraro 1995; Warr 2000). However, the idea that fear of crime is entirely "irrational" and driven purely by emotion has been refuted by scholars (Gabriel and Greve 2003; Jackson 2005). For example, Jackson (2005) argues that fear of crime involves a complex interplay of cognitive, emotional, behavioural, and social processes. He asserts that fear of crime consists of worry associated with specific events, subjective risk perceptions, and an assessment or interpretation of the social and physical environment. Worry, rather than anxiety or fear is used in his definition as worry encompasses the transitory nature of experiences with crime and disorder, whereas fear is too broad and may capture more profuse concerns about a range of social problems (Gabriel and Greve 2003; Gromet and Pronin 2009).

Another key element of Jackson's definition is that an individual's fear of crime is directly influenced by subjective probabilities of crime risk. Research across a number of disciplines has found that instead of assessing the mathematical probabilities of an event occurring, people tend to assess the *subjective probabilities* of an event occurring (Windschitl 2002). These subjective probabilities of risk are influenced by internal and external forces that are sometimes irrelevant to an individual's actual risk (Windschitl 2002). Furthermore, research demonstrates that several subjective factors (such as context, beliefs and environmental cues) play a significant role in whether people consider a risk to be high or low (Mishra et al. 2009). In the case of fear of crime, fear may not be fuelled entirely by an individual's emotional state, but rather faulty cognitions that are incongruent with an individual's actual likelihood or risk of crime victimisation (Farrall et al. 1997; Farrall and Gadd 2004; Jackson 2004; Hale 1996).

Finally, Jackson's definition of fear of crime considers how individuals' perceptions of the environment may influence their worry about crime victimisation. He argues that environments characterised by high amounts of disorganisation and disorderly behaviour from community members may produce concerns of imminent crime risk and in turn increase an individual's fear of crime (Jackson 2005). This is further mediated by social processes within neighbourhoods that may serve as a protective buffer against victimisation concerns, such as individuals' perceptions of social cohesion and perceptions of informal social control in an area (Brunton-Smith and Sturgis 2011; Chataway and Hart 2016; Chataway et al. 2017; Jackson 2004).

Based on the aforementioned work that has attempted to define and operationalise the various components that may contribute to fearing crime, we propose that definitions of fear of crime aim to capture the construct as a social-psychological process, rather than constraining definitions to focus only on emotional elements of fear. In other words, definitions of fear of crime should tap into its affective (i.e., worry, dread, anxiety), behavioural (i.e., precautionary behaviour) and cognitive features (i.e., risk perceptions). Definitions should consider that these affective, behavioural and cognitive features of fear may be further mediated by specific characteristics of the physical and social environment that have the potential to elicit concern about crime victimisations. Therefore, we propose that fear of crime be defined as: *an affective, behavioural and cognitive response to signals or cues of out of character behaviour that come to symbolise crime and the degradation of community values and social order* (Gabriel and Greve 2003; Garofalo and Laub 1978; Innes 2004; Jackson 2004).

7.2 Measuring Fear of Crime, Perceptions of Disorder, and Quality of Life

In addition to debates around the 'meaning' of fear of crime, there has also been a number of attempts to refine the measurement of the construct over recent years. Scholars have utilised a number of methods to evaluate fear of crime, perceptions of disorder, and quality of life in neighbourhoods and public spaces. The bulk of literature uses the terms *disorder* and *incivilities* interchangeably, and throughout this chapter our focus is on disorder and incivilities which occur within the neighbourhood context. LaGrange et al. (1992) captures the general consensus of what constitutes neighbourhood disorder and incivilities—that is, incivilities are considered to be "low level breaches of community standards that signal an erosion of conventionally accepted norms and values" (p. 312). It is important to note that whilst incivilities can be criminal actions, this is not always necessarily the case. For example, non-criminal types of incivilities used by LaGrange et al. (1992) include the presence of litter and inconsiderate neighbours.

One of the most commonly used methods of establishing baselines of fear of crime and neighbourhood disorder within the community are surveys (Hale 1996; Farrall and Gadd 2004; Lee and Mythen 2018). In contrast to surveys, qualitative approaches such as observations, interviews, and focus groups have been used to understand the lived experiences of individuals in their neighbourhoods and their subsequent interactions with crime and local disorder. These qualitative approaches allow for a deeper level understanding of the socio-political and community-level causes of fear of crime and disorder (Lee 2013; Lupton and Tulloch 1999). However, the survey (in paper-pencil and online forms) remains the most common tool used to evaluate fear of crime and perceptions of disorder within the scholarly literature, due to the cost effectiveness of administering surveys and the ability to generalise survey findings to the broader population.

Although there are a number of benefits to using surveys to collect information about fear of crime, some scholars have argued that survey research on fear of crime has the capacity to produce/invent the very problem it seeks to measure (Lee 2013). Lee, in his seminal book *Inventing Fear of Crime*, tracks the politicisation of fear of crime, arguing that the concept was rarely ever used as an organising principle in criminological and political discourse prior to the 1960s, and that researchers, through the use of surveys, potentially created the concept of fear of crime. He argues that the measurement of fear of crime in early household surveys indicated significantly high levels of fear, resulting in fear of crime becoming a "social problem" that required immediate governmental action. Although, as you will see below, the idea that fear of crime was on the rise in communities may be the product of how it was measured in these early surveys, rather than the politicisation and emergence of "fear of crime" in criminological discourse.

Historically, measures of fear of crime can be traced back to household surveys conducted in the United States in the 1960s (Biderman et al. 1967; Ennis 1967; Reiss 1967). These national surveys aimed to obtain accurate statistics about the level of crime victimisation experienced in various cities in the US, along with providing information about people's beliefs and attitudes towards crime, safety, policing, and punishment (Lee 2007). Similarly, in the United Kingdom, a number of sweeps of the British Crime Survey (now the Crime Survey for England and Wales) contained questions on not only crime victimisation, but also fear of crime and perceptions of victimisation risk. These national surveys are further supplemented by local crime surveys aimed to measure levels of fear of crime within smaller geographic areas (see for example, Anderson et al. 1990; Chataway and Hart 2016; Crawford et al. 1990; Last and Jackson 1988; Mawby 1986).

Global measures of fear of crime. Early surveys used to evaluate the prevalence of fear of crime in the community tended to rely on what Garofalo (1981) refers to as "global measures" of safety. Perceptions of safety questions have been regarded as the "defacto gold standard" for measuring fear of crime for a number of years (Warr 2000), and have included question items such as:

- How safe do you feel being out alone in your neighbourhood or area after dark?
- How safe would you feel being out alone in your neighbourhood or area after dark?
- Is there any place around here where you feel unsafe walking at night?

Unfortunately, these types of questions do not mention crime specifically, limiting the generalisability of responses to specific crime threats or disorderly environments (i.e., personal victimisation) (Hale 1996). These questions also do not provide a clear geographic or temporal reference point for respondents, and instead focus on rather broad geographic areas such as the respondent's "neighbourhood" or "area", thereby ignoring individual's perceptions of safety in public spaces outside of these familiar environments (Garofalo and Laub 1978; Skogan 1981). This is important in the context of criminal victimisation, because crime is influenced by opportunity, but opportunities to commit offences are not distributed evenly across time and space (Hart and Lersch 2015). The same principle applies to fear of crime, as fear of crime is not evenly distributed within space and time, and exposure to events that elicit crime concern are considered to be context-dependent or transitory (Fisher and Nasar 1992; Chataway et al. 2017; Solymosi et al. 2015). Finally, these questions describe situations that are hypothetical and may not represent realistic behaviours that all members of the public engage in (Hale 1996). For example, elderly individuals are less likely to venture outside at night alone, for a number of reasons other than crime. Moreover, the physical effects of aging and mobility decline may lead to higher risk of a fall at night when visual acuity is low, and therefore elderly individuals may choose not to walk alone at night due to these health—but not—crime related risks (Tsai et al. 2016).

Summary and intensity of victimisation questions. Due to these criticisms of perceptions of safety questions, further refinements in the measurement of fear of crime have resulted in surveys that ask respondents to summarise their levels of worry about specific types of crimes (e.g., property offences), their likelihood of victimisation, and their intensity of such feelings and experiences (Farrall et al. 1997; Farrall and Gadd 2004; Jackson 2005). These types of questions allow researchers to identify qualitative differences between fear of specific forms of crime; and measure risk perception or one's perception of imminent danger or threat.

Although more specific in wording, these types of questions still mask complex processes associated with fearing crime (Farrall et al. 1997; Jackson 2005). For example, Jackson (2005) asserts that fear may generate a variety of emotions associated with crime, such as, worry, anger, and hostility about potential risk of victimisation. These emotions may be persistent low-level states or specific reactions to crime that are associated with a specific threat in one's immediate environment (Gabriel and Greve 2003). Moreover, questions that focus on the intensity of emotional experiences with crime regard these emotions as rigid and enduring, rather than experiences that vary in time and are only expressed when in a particular place or location (Gabriel and Greve 2003; Gray et al. 2008; Solymosi et al. 2015).

Frequency questions and fear of crime. To address some of these concerns with intensity questions, contemporary surveys examining fear of crime tend to utilise frequency questions. Frequency questions ask respondents to reflect back on a short period of time (usually a month) and count how often they have felt worried or fearful about falling victim to a specific crime or form of victimisation (Farrall et al. 1997; Jackson 2005). These questions are temporally specific (e.g., over a month, a day) and provide information about the frequency and extent of experiences of worry about crime (Tseloni and Zarafonitou 2008). They can also be tailored to the individual's own neighbourhood, allowing researchers to identify any background concerns (i.e., disorder) in relation to crime fear. However, concerns around precision and the ecological validity of frequency questions have been raised by some scholars (see for example, Chataway et al. 2019; Solymosi et al. 2015).

In particular, concerns centre on the retrospective wording of frequency questions: "*how often have you worried about becoming the victim of a crime over the last month in this area?*" with scholars arguing that these questions treat fear of crime as a static construct (Solymosi et al. 2015). As a result, surveys using retrospective frequency questions, cannot resolve challenges associated with situating and contextualising fear of crime in the proximate environment. Moreover, asking individuals to reflect back on past experiences of worry about crime, may lead to misinterpretations of past events due to human memory decay and individual cognitive capacities, especially when survey data is collected using cross-sectional methods (Gazzaniga et al. 2011). Some events may be represented more saliently (or proximal) by an individual and restrict their ability to recall all relevant experiences of crime victimisation over a long period of time such as a month. Alternatively, some events may be considered to be more distal, than they actually are in one's environment, and result in an under-estimation of fear of crime.

To summarise, numerous methods have been used to capture fear of crime within neighbourhood environments with varying success. Despite improvements to the way we measure fear of crime and its related constructs such as perceptions of disorder, their remains concerns around how the construct can be measured and positioned within the proximate environment, given the context-dependent nature of crime, disorder, and fear of crime. As you will see in a later section of this Chapter, researchers are currently piloting new methods for capturing fear of crime and perceptions of disorder when they are experienced within an individual's proximate environment. These new methods may address many of the concerns raised with traditional survey instruments designed to measure fear of crime and localised disorder.

7.3 Correlates of Fear of Crime

Up until this point we have described how fear of crime emerged as a topic of scientific enquiry, how it has been operationalised and measured in past studies, and some of the existing challenges associated with common tools used to examine fear of crime and related constructs such as neighbourhood disorder. Below, we describe some of the key theoretical hypotheses and known determinants of fear of crime, that have been discovered using the methods/measures discussed above.

Individual-Level Correlates of Fear. Numerous theoretical correlates of fear of crime have been identified. Contemporary research tends to categorise these into individual, situational and social predictors. Common individual correlates of fear of crime include gender, age, education, and marital status. Gender is one of the most significant demographic predictors of fear of crime (Franklin et al. 2008; Liu et al. 2009; McCrea et al. 2005). Moreover, researchers have identified that women consistently report higher levels of fear of crime in comparison to men (Abdullah et al. 2014; Callanan and Teasdale 2009; Cops and Pleysier 2010; Chataway and Hart 2018). In particular, women tend to report higher levels of worry and fear of becoming a victim of personal crime, despite being less likely to become the victims of this type of crime in comparison to men (Ferraro 1995; Gray et al. 2008).

Individuals age, education, and marital status have also been found to be correlated with fear of crime to varying extents. Much of the available literature suggests that the elderly tend to be more fearful of crime than their younger counterparts (e.g. Braungart et al. 1980; Clemente and Kleiman 1977; Fox et al. 2009; LaGrange and Ferraro 1989; Lee 1983; Ollenburger 1981). This is despite the fact that elderly people are generally at a far lower risk of encountering victimisation (Garofalo and Laub 1978). The demographic variables of education and marital status are less consistently related to fear of crime, although some research suggests that those who are less educated are more fearful than those with higher levels of education (Clemente and Kleiman 1977; Covington and Taylor 1991; Gibson et al. 2002), and individuals who are not married are more fearful than those who are married (Braungart et al. 1980; Keane 1998; Toseland 1982; Will and McGrath 1995).

Over the years, researchers have attempted to explore individual differences in fear of crime, through the application of various models and hypotheses. One hypothesis that has been used to explain individual differences in fear of crime is the Differential Vulnerability Hypothesis (Cops and Pleysier 2010). According to this hypothesis, those who are more socially or physically vulnerable are expected to report higher levels of fear of crime (Liu et al. 2009; Rader et al. 2012). The traditional view of the vulnerability hypothesis was that the disproportionate amount of fear of crime reported among women and the elderly was related to their heightened perceptions of personal vulnerability (Hale 1996; LaGrange and Ferraro 1989; Stanko 1995). However, this view has recently fallen out of favour among scholars due to a lack of research into what actually constitutes "personal" vulnerability (Callanan and Teasdale 2009).

Due to this, researchers have developed alternative explanations for individual differences in fear of crime. For example, Warr (1984) asserts that an important concept for understanding individual differences in fear of crime is risk sensitivity. According to the risk sensitivity model, a perceived level of risk is needed to elicit fear of crime if the consequences of crime are judged to be serious. In the case of gender and fear of crime, it is argued that women are more sensitive to the consequences of victimisation than men and commonly report lower levels of perceived self-efficacy or control over crime (Warr 1984, 1990). The same pattern is also observed among age and fear of crime, with elderly individuals being more sensitive to crime risks than younger individuals (Killias 1990).

Empirical evidence in support of Warr's (1990) risk sensitivity model has been offered by Jackson (2009), who found that women tended to worry more about personal crimes than men in a sample of UK residents. He also documented that women felt less in control of becoming the victim of crime. Consequently, women rated the likelihood and consequences of victimisation as being higher than men. These findings suggest that women tend to be more sensitive to personal crimes and report lower levels of control over potential victimisation in line with Warr's risk sensitivity model. Contrary to the work described above, contemporary research suggests that the ways in which men and women think about crime are actually quite similar (Chataway and Hart 2018). Chataway and Hart (2018) found that risk perception tends to play an important role in the development of worry about personal and property-based victimisation among both Australian men and women. They found that perceptions of the social and physical environment (i.e., perceptions of neighbourhood disorder) had a more significant impact on risk sensitivity among men in their sample of Australian residents, suggesting that the context (the perceived amount of disorder in an area) in which attitudes about crime are expressed plays an important role in eliciting concern about crime victimisation for men.

7.4 Situational Level Correlates of Fear

Whereas vulnerability models focus on individual "proxy" factors that affect perceptions of risk, neighbourhood and disorder models emphasise the importance of the immediate environment on an individual's fear of crime. Proponents of these models argue that in order to understand how fear of crime varies among individuals, we must assess the influence of local community characteristics and neighbourhood-level social processes (Brunton-Smith and Sturgis 2011). In particular, research stemming from these models assesses the effect of social disorganisation on informal social control mechanisms in the community and how disorganisation and decay in neighbourhoods may produce fear of crime. The physical and social environment can also signal to residents the state of a neighbourhood and its levels of community health, along with the potential for victimisation to occur (Box et al. 1988; Ferraro 1995; Skogan 1990; Taylor 2001; Wilson and Kelling 1982; Weisburd and White 2019).

The basic premise of neighbourhood models is that fear and anxiety about crime are a consequence of the wider social environment in which crime occurs (Ferraro 1995). According to Brunton-Smith and Sturgis (2011), there are four principle mechanisms through which neighbourhoods may influence fear: (a) through rational responses to variability across neighbourhoods in the incidence of crime; (b) the organisational structure of neighbourhoods that promote or inhibit collective efficacy and social cohesion; (c) through visual signs of disorder, both social and physical in nature; and (d) through the moderating effects of neighbourhood-level characteristics on individual-level causes of fear. These themes identified by Brunton-Smith and Sturgis (2011) are consistently reported across many studies exploring the effects of neighbourhood conditions on resident's concerns of crime victimisation (see for example; Chataway and Hart 2016; Corcoran et al. 2018; Herbert 1993).

Socio-economic Composition of Neighbourhoods and Fear of Crime. Early research exploring the relationship between neighbourhoods, crime, and fear of crime hypothesised that the socioeconomic composition of a neighbourhood may encourage or discourage offending behaviour (Brunton-Smith and Sturgis 2011). For example, individuals who live in low socio-economic neighbourhoods may have limited access to materials goods and services, and therefore may have a greater incentive to obtain such goods through illegitimate means (robbery and theft). It is argued that the incidence of these types of crimes will be greater in neighbourhoods containing a large number of individuals who do not have access to the financial capital necessary for survival (Brunton-Smith and Sturgis 2011). If residents respond rationally to crime risks, then it is argued that those living in less affluent areas should report greater levels of fear of crime, in comparison to those living in more affluent areas. In this case, fear of crime is considered a rational response to the actual crime risks present in the neighbourhood in which an individual lives (Brunton-Smith and Sturgis 2011; Jackson 2005).

However, limited evidence has found significant links between neighbourhood crime rates and fear of crime. Moreover, some researchers have identified that there is no association between fear of crime and actual victimisation, leading them to speculate that fear of crime is more so related to subjective markers (i.e., perceptions of incivility) in the physical environment (Ferraro 1995). In contrast to these views, some studies have found weak associations between fear of crime and local crime rates. For example, a study by Liska et al. (1982) found that in cities that had higher rates of recorded crime, residents were more likely to have higher levels of fear, when controlling for specific characteristics of each city. Taylor (2001) also found a weak relationship between fear of crime and recorded property crime in Baltimore, after controlling for signals of disorder and other structural characteristics of neighbourhoods. However, both studies are limited in terms of their generalisability to the broader population and analytic procedures utilising aggregate-level analyses.

Other studies have explored interactions between specific measures of socioeconomic status (i.e., access to education) and individual variables such as gender and age and have documented significant relationships with fear of crime. For example, Mesch (2000) found that Israeli women's fear of crime could be explained by their level of income and levels of educational attainment (both of which are proxy measures of SES). That is, women who had low levels of personal income and limited access to education, were more likely to fear crime, than those who were educated and had more stable personal income. However, Mesch notes that these findings of a link between SES and fear of crime should be cautioned as other measures of socioeconomic status such as household density and household size did not significantly predict Israeli women's fear of crime.

Structural Characteristics of Neighbourhoods and Fear of Crime. Neighbourhoods can also influence perceptions of crime through structural components of the built environment. The structure of the built environment has been found to be an important predictor of low-level disorder and crime (Shaw and McKay 1942). Shaw and McKay (1942) are often credited for their extensive analysis of structural characteristics of neighbourhoods and their effect on juvenile delinquency in Chicago neighbourhoods. This macro-level sociological theory postulates that neighbourhood structural factors inhibit a community's ability to self-regulate, which in turn leads to crime and delinquency (Chataway et al. 2017; Park and Burgess 1924).

According to Shaw and McKay (1942), there are three structural characteristics of neighbourhoods that are important for explaining crime experienced within neighbourhoods. These are: (a) neighbourhood socioeconomic status; (b) residential mobility; and (c) ethnic heterogeneity. Specifically, rapid population growth within low socioeconomic and ethnically heterogeneous neighbourhoods may lead to a breakdown in both formal and informal social norms (Shaw and McKay 1942). This breakdown limits the capacity of residents to control outsiders from committing illegal or socially disruptive behaviours within their neighbourhoods (Brunton-Smith and Sturgis 2011).

Contemporary research by Sampson and Raudenbush (2001) has found that the social and organisational characteristics and processes of neighbourhoods can undermine other community level processes such as collective efficacy. This in turn leads to a greater prevalence of neighbourhood disorder and criminal activity in areas with low levels of collective efficacy. Sampson (2009) also notes that neighbourhood structural characteristics often act as cues of deficient social control mechanisms, which may exaggerate, and distort subjective perceptions of the prevalence of disorder in an area. Moreover, these ideas about social disorganisation and collective efficacy have theoretical relevance to fear of crime. Neighbourhood social-structural change is thought to affect fear of crime through both direct and indirect means. For example, social-structural change may increase offending and disorderly behaviour in a neighbourhood, along with signalling the deterioration of community health, standards, social control, and efficacy (Brunton-Smith and Sturgis 2011; Sampson and Raudenbush 2001; Sampson 2009).

In contrast to limited and inconsistent findings on reported rates of neighbourhood crime and fear, research on the effects of neighbourhood structural and organisational characteristics has identified stronger links with fear of crime. Specifically, researchers have identified significant associations between fear of crime in inner city areas (characterised by high population density) when compared to urban and rural communities, supporting Shaw and McKay's theory of social disorganisation (see Allen 2006; Killias 1990). Other scholars have found that individuals living in large ethnically heterogeneous communities are more fearful of crime than those in less ethnically diverse communities (see Covington and Taylor 1991; Lane and Meeker 2000).

Disorderly Environments and Fear of Crime. Another argument within the criminological literature is that disorderly neighbourhood characteristics can influence fear, beyond an individual's actual level of crime risk (Brunton-Smith and Sturgis 2011). This idea proposes that visible signs of disorder can distort or cloud an individual's perception of crime risk; and as a result, increase their fear of crime. Wilson and Kelling (1982) expanded on Shaw and McKay's work on socio-structural characteristics of neighbourhoods and crime, by introducing the broken windows thesis to the literature on neighbourhood disorder. Specifically, Wilson and Kelling (1982) argued that when physical and social disorder is left untreated in an area or neighbourhood, it can be indicative of a more serious social problem, such as the physical breakdown of informal social control mechanisms in a neighbourhood. The broken windows thesis has influenced a number of policy frameworks and programs since its inception, given its common-sense appeal, and positive findings from the application of broken windows style policing in New York City in the 1990s (see Innes 2004; Skogan 1990).

An extensive body of literature has been devoted to defining disorder, along with qualitatively categorising disorder. The definition utilised by LaGrange et al. (1992) which was explained earlier in this Chapter captures the general consensus of what incivility and disorder constitutes within the neighbourhood context. LaGrange et al. (1992) included in their definition of incivility disordered *physical* environments (i.e., neighbourhoods/public places characterised by graffiti, litter/rubbish, abandoned vehicles, and dilapidated buildings), and disorderly/disruptive *social* conditions (i.e., public drunkenness, rowdy/unruly youth, open drug taking, and inconsiderate neighbours). This operationalisation of incivility mirrors early work evaluating disorder perceptions in US neighbourhoods by Hunter (1978). Hunter identified a range of low-level signs of disorder such as vandalism, graffiti, deteriorated dwellings, unsupervised teenage groups, and litter, that were synonymous with environments prone to the potential for crime. Hunter argued that these visible cues provide residents with information about the extent to which a neighbourhood is in decline; and therefore, unable to exercise the social control necessary to prevent crime and disorderly behaviour.

More contemporary research expanding on this early work suggests that physical disorder can be separated from physical decay (Sampson 2009; Sampson and Raudenbush 1999, 2004). Put simply, physical disorder is the result of specific destructive behaviour (e.g., graffiti); whilst physical decay arises from a potential lack of institutional investment in an area, which results in structural changes to an environment (e.g., abandoned buildings, deteriorated dwellings) (Grubesic et al. 2018; Sampson 2009).

It is important to note that the above definitions of incivility exclude serious criminal violations or infractions, such as rape, armed robbery, and assault. However, some contemporary evidence suggests individuals' abilities to differentiate low-level incivility from crime is dependent on the socio-economic composition of neighbourhoods (Cheshire and Fitzgerald 2015). Despite this, we have chosen to distinguish between serious crime/criminal violations and low-level breaches that may not necessarily carry criminal sanctions but are nonetheless perceived by residents as a signal of community decline and deterioration of informal social control mechanisms within neighbourhoods.

Signals of disorder can often be more important determinants of fear of crime than reported crime rates in a neighbourhood. Hunter (1978) asserts that such signs of disorder are readily visible in communities and can capture a broad range of signals of community decline in comparison to official crime statistics. However, visual signs of disorder are difficult to quantify, and most researchers rely on self-report measures of disorder rather than independently collecting information about disorder through observational or street auditing methods (Brunton-Smith and Sturgis 2011). Brunton-Smith and Sturgis (2011) highlight that "this strategy leaves open the possibility that any observed effect of disorder on fear of crime is endogenous, with fear of crime driving perceptions of disorder rather than (or in addition to) the other way around" (p. 338).

Another difficulty with the measurement of disorder is that most studies are context specific. This is problematic because cues of disorder may be represented differently across multiple locations and may be culturally derived. Spelman (2004) argues that if different forms of incivility induce fear of crime, and other reactions in different contexts, then indices of incivility may not capture the full extent of subjective cues in the environment that come to represent disorder for an individual. For example, recent empirical work analysing "fix my street" data (a reporting system where residents report local problems) in the United Kingdom found that reports of disorder vary across environments and across time of day, with some incivilities more frequently reported in specific areas than others (Solymosi et al. 2017). Moreover, Solymosi and her colleagues found that residents reported incivilities that they encountered through the use of a particular space. These incivilities served as signs of disorderly behaviour that had occurred in the area during the previous day and that were encountered by residents during their everyday routine activities (i.e., broken bottles, litter, rats, dead animals).

Leading on from the issues above, Worrall (2006) argues that there are three core methodological problems with the incivility thesis (or model). Firstly, as previously described, there is currently no clear number of incivility or disorder indicators within the literature. Secondly, researchers utilise a variety of methods to measure the prevalence of incivility, which often result in inconsistent findings. For example, Piquero (1999) found that on-site assessments of incivility in an area were different from incivility estimates using self-report survey measures. Lastly, some researchers have argued that the prevalence of incivility may not be separable from estimates of the prevalence of related constructs, such as criminal victimisation. This poses the question of whether individuals are capable of separating incivility (or low-level breaches of community standards) from crime (Worrall 2006).

Nevertheless, numerous large-scale neighbourhood studies have identified how disorder and fear of crime are intertwined. For example, a study by Markowitz et al. (2001) assessed neighbourhood data collected from the British Crime Survey (BCS) and found that disorder had a significant effect on individuals' perceptions of crime. Interestingly, Markowitz et al. (2001) identified that perceptions of disorder can feedback into increasing the prevalence disorder in the community. Moreover, when controlling neighborhood crime rates, the authors found that disorder had a more significant impact on fear of crime than actual reported incidents of crime. Similarly, investigations in Australia have identified perceptions of disorder to be the most significant predictor of fear of crime, when controlling for socio-demographic variables. McCrea et al. (2005) assessed fear of crime in a sample of Brisbane residents and found that perceptions of disorder were the most significant predictor of fear of crime. In particular, physical signs of disorder such as graffiti were identified to have the most significant association with perceptions of unsafe environments at night.

More contemporary theoretical perspectives such as the signals crime perspective (SCP) have been developed to further describe the link between disorder and victimisation risk. Innes (2004) defines a signal crime as a "criminal incident that is interpreted as indicating the presence of criminogenic risk." (p. 350). Signals of disorder are denoted by physical and social cues within the environment, which in turn shape risk perceptions. He also describes two other types of signals related to fear of crime—control signals and signal events. Control signals relate to communication between individuals about social control actions underway in neighbourhoods, which are believed to moderate and shape individuals' perceptions of risk. On the other hand, signal events relate to immediate incidents that are not defined by legal conventions as "crimes" but nevertheless may signal community decline and in turn shape risk perceptions (Innes 2004). The basic premise of the SCP is that some types of crime may amplify individuals' levels of perceived crime risk, while others may not. This amplified risk produces possible affective (i.e., feelings of concern in relation to specific types of crime) and behavioural responses (i.e., avoidance of a particular place). At present, evaluations of SCP to fear of crime have been restricted to qualitative methodologies and small samples (Innes 2004). Thus, more empirical work is needed to determine whether individuals represent disorder in respect to the four distinct signals outlined by Innes (2004).

Interactions Between Individual and Situational Level Correlates of Fear. As mentioned previously, structural and physical characteristics of the neighbourhood can have a direct effect on reported levels of fear of crime. However, another important area of research on neighbourhoods and fear of crime centres around the moderating effect of neighbourhoods on individual-level causes of crime and fear. In other words, an individual-level characteristic (i.e., gender) that shapes an individual's perception of crime risk may operate differently as a function of the neighbourhood in which they live (Brunton-Smith and Sturgis 2011; Solymosi et al. 2015). Empirical work does support moderating effects between disorder, individual-level variables and fear of crime. For example, McGarrell et al. (1997) found that individual differences in fear of crime, varied as a function of low-level disorder in the community. Specifically, in areas where high levels of disorder were absent, individual level characteristics were highly predictive of one's fear of crime. However, when neighbourhoods were characterised by high levels of disorder, this difference was less apparent.

In other research, Taylor et al. (1985), found that social class moderated the relationship between disorder and fear of crime. Specifically, Taylor et al. (1985) identified that blue-collar workers were significantly more sensitive to visual cues of disorder, than poor or more affluent individuals. According to Taylor et al., poor individuals were more concerned with immediate threats of danger in the environment. Whereas, affluent individuals, regarded signals of disorder as transitory, and not stable attributes or reflections of the area. A more recent study by Snedker (2015) examined the relationship between neighbourhood disorder, gender and fear of crime. Snedker found that although there was no variability in perceptions of disorder in a neighbourhood (between men and women), the reaction to incivility differed amongst genders. Specifically, Snedker found that two types of neighbourhood conditions (physical disorder and serious violent crime) help to explain greater levels of fear of crime reported by women in their neighbourhoods. The overall finding of this study was that women who perceived greater neighbourhood risks were more likely to fall in higher fear of crime categories. These findings demonstrate that the differential impacts of neighbourhood conditions on fear of crime may also help to explain gender differences in fear of crime. Furthermore, the findings suggest that women's fear may be related to a sense of ecological vulnerability (Snedker 2015). Although the above studies do suggest that there is a moderating effect of disorder on individual level characteristics that in turn shape fear, their self-reported data collection methods make it difficult to determine whether fear of crime drives perceptions of disorder, or whether this relationship is reversed with disorder driving fear of crime and perceptions of crime risk (Brunton-Smith and Sturgis 2011).

7.5 Social Processes: Social Integration Models of Crime Fear

Social integration, social capital, and crime fear. Social integration models are also another type of model used to explain fear of crime. Generally, the work stemming from this position is based on two qualitatively different, but theoretically similar constructs of social capital and social control. Social capital refers to "features of social organisation such as networks, norms, and social trust that facilitate coordination and cooperation for mutual benefit" (Putnam 1995, p. 67). According to Agnew (1995) those who are involved in social support networks can enhance their access to information and human or material resources; this may in turn decrease the onset of criminal victimisation. Similarly, high levels of social support are perceived to be beneficial for adopting self-protective behaviours in response to crime (Ferguson and Mindel 2007).

However, mixed findings are reported in studies assessing the relationship between social features of neighbourhoods and fear of crime (Ferguson and Mindel 2007). For example, Thompson and Krause (1998) found that levels of connection (embeddedness) in social support networks had no effect in reducing resident's levels of anxiety associated with crime, in crime prone neighbourhoods. Moreover, Sacco (1993) found that participation in social networks in a neighbourhood actually increased individual's feelings of anxiety associated with crime and potential victimisation experience. Other researchers have found a positive effect of social capital and integration on fear of crime. For example, Rountree and Land (1996) found that social integration with one's neighbours diminishes perceptions of danger and threat. Moreover, Lewis and Salem (1986) found that fear of crime was low in neighbourhoods in which neighbours had well developed social ties with one another, demonstrating the importance of social bonds and connections.

Informal social control and crime fear. Social control is another important construct of the social integration models, and has been argued as an important predictor of fear of crime. In one of the first studies to be conducted on fear of crime, Biderman et al. (1967) identified that increasing levels of crime in an area come to represent a threat to order and cohesion. These crimes evoke intense public reactions to punishment and can be taken as a sign of threat to the moral order (Biderman et al. 1967). Alternatively, crime results in mistrust of both those who are formally responsible for maintaining social order (e.g., the police and local authorities), and informally responsible for maintaining connections and order (e.g., neighbours) (Ross and Jang 2000).

Moreover, ties formed by individuals within a neighbourhood are perceived as necessary in order to transmit behavioural expectations and informal sanctions when such ties are violated (Warner and Rountree 1997). Furthermore, it is through these ties in which common norms and rules are articulated and informal sanctions (for disruptive behaviours that are against the moral order) are carried out (Warner and Rountree 1997). Therefore, it is believed that communities with wider friendships and social ties have a greater capacity to exercise informal social control, which in turn reduces fear of crime (Warner and Rountree 1997). In reference to the effect of social control on fear of crime, research has identified neighbourhoods that exercise informal social control methods are less fearful of crime. In a study conducted by Gainey et al. (2011), residents who perceived that their community had lost control over crime and disorder were more likely to fear crime. This research supports the notion that social control plays a pertinent role in predicting fear of crime.

Converging models of fear of crime. Existing models of fear of crime usually (with exception to qualitative methodologies) apply an assortment of multivariate techniques to a variety of psychological and sociological predictors of fear of crime, in an attempt to create ad hoc models of crime fear (Van der Wurrf et al. 1989). These ad hoc models only capture the influence of psychological and sociological variables within isolation, and therefore limit a researcher's ability to examine the mediational processes associated with the development of fear of crime and related constructs such as perceptions of disorder. In an attempt to synthesise the existing fear of crime scholarship, Jackson (2005) has developed and tested an alternative theoretical model of crime fear that accounts for how fear of crime consists of worry associated with specific events, subjective risk perceptions, and an assessment of the social and physical environment. Jackson refers to this model as a *Social-Psychological Model of Victimisation Worry*.

The model assumes that there are five unique dimensions of fear of crime; each dimension is based on the research mentioned above that tests vulnerability, neighbourhood and social integration models of fear of crime. The five dimensions are (a) frequency of *worry* about crime; (b) perceived *likelihood* of crime; (c) perceived *consequences* crime; (d) perceived *control* over crime; and (e) *beliefs* about the incidence of crime. Included within the model are perceptions of the environment, namely *incivility* and *social cohesion*. The model is presented in Fig. 7.1.

According to Jackson (2004, 2005), each dimension of the model aims to capture the social-psychological processes that characterise worry about crime. Jackson and other researchers have undertaken numerous reliability assessments of his social psychological model (Chataway and Hart 2016, 2018; Chataway et al. 2019; Jackson 2004, 2005, 2009). The first reliability study of Jackson's model tested the new dimensions of victimisation worry using a large representative sample of London residents. Jackson collected data using a mail survey of 1800 adults in two socio-economically contrasting areas of London (Jackson 2005). A total of 479 completed questionnaires were returned. Using Confirmatory Factor Analysis (CFA) to assess the overall reliability and validity of the measures, Jackson identified that a two-factor model based on crime type (i.e., personal and property crime) fitted the data better than a one-factor model that assessed each individual indicator of crime.

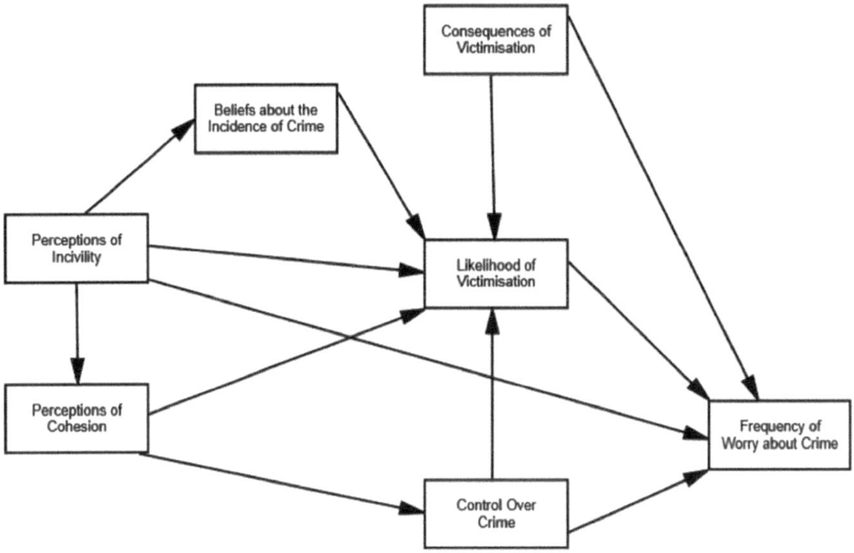

Fig. 7.1 Jackson's (2005) social-psychological process model of victimisation worry

Confirmatory factor analyses identified that participants thought about crime in different ways. For example, being the victim of a personal crime was not the same as being a victim of a property offence. Secondly, in relation to the five proposed constructs of the model, Jackson found that all constructs had good scaling properties. In addition to this finding, participants regarded *worry*, perceived *likelihood*, perceived *control*, perceived *consequences*, and *beliefs* about crime as separate constructs (Jackson 2005). In other words, perceived likelihood of victimisation was not the same as perceived consequences of victimisation.

A five-factor model fitted the data better than both a four-factor model that combined worry and likelihood, and a three-factor model that combined likelihood, control and consequences to reflect risk appraisal or perception. Subsequently, these findings indicated that the five constructs are empirically distinct from each other, demonstrating discriminant validity (Jackson 2005). Thus, all five constructs measured different facets or dimensions of fear of crime. In relation to the impact of the social and physical environment, existing studies indicate that both incivility and social cohesion measures demonstrate significant reliability and validity, according to model fit indices. Moreover, results indicated that perceptions of the environment shaped participants overall assessment of the incidence of crime, personal threat and vulnerability (Jackson 2005). The reliability of this model has also been assessed and similar results replicated in the Australian context (Chataway and Hart 2016, 2018).

To summarise, there are numerous models designed to better understand how fear of crime arises within neighbourhoods and public spaces. These models tend to focus on *individual-level* variables such as vulnerability gender and age, *environmental characteristics* such as socioeconomic status, social disorganisation, and disorder perceptions, and *social characteristics* of environments such as social capital and informal social control. Despite a growing understanding of the correlates that produce fear of crime, issues remain with respect to how these models are tested and conceptualised, and in particular, the use of regression techniques to generate ad hoc models of fear of crime. Attempts have been made to simplify these fear of crime models, by considering the interactions between vulnerability/risk perception, perceptions of the immediate physical and social environment, and worry or concern about crime. Studies testing these social-psychological models of victimisation worry have demonstrated that fear of crime can be considered as a process related to specific dimensions of worry, likelihood, consequences, control, and belief. These dimensions are further influenced by an individual's assessments of the physical and social environment around them.

7.6 New Developments in the Study of Fear of Crime, Disorder and Quality of Life

Ecological momentary assessments of fear and disorder perceptions. As mentioned previously, new methodologies are currently being tested to better capture perceptions of crime and disorder in the proximate environment, signalling a shift in our empirical understanding of fear of crime as a series of experiences or "remembered events" that occur in the past, to an event that occurs within the proximate environment of an individual. These new methodologies are referred to as Ecological Momentary Assessments or Ambulatory Assessments and are used to capture social behaviour as it occurs in the real world using innovative data collection tools such as smartphones (Shiffman 2009).

In recent years, scholars have attempted to use smartphone technology to collect information about context-dependent fear of crime and immediate perceptions of neighbourhood disorder/incivilities (see Chataway et al. 2017; Solymosi et al. 2015). Recently, Chataway et al. (2019) used a commercial smartphone application called MetricWire to develop and test a new momentary model of victimisation worry adapted from Jackson (2005) that considers how immediate perceptions of disorder are intertwined with transitory experiences of crime risk and worry towards particular types of crime. They found that immediate perceptions of disorder (as measured by physical and social indicators of disorder) predict an individual's immediate assessment of crime risk, which in turn influences worry/concern about personal victimisation in one's proximate environment. Moreover, signs of physical and social disorder in the immediate environment were found to directly increase an individual's level of risk sensitivity in the immediate area. When risk sensitivity was high an increase in momentary worry about crime was also observed using the new momentary model. This study provides a new avenue for assessing perceptions of crime and local disorder within the immediate environment using a new momentary model (provided below). These methods are important in general, as they allow scholars to better contextualise and situate fear of crime and specific neighbourhood problems/disorder (Solymosi et al. 2015; Chataway et al. 2017).

Chataway et al. (2019) suggest that new interventions can now potentially be developed to target specific dimensions of their momentary model of victimisation worry. For example, information campaigns challenging misconceptions about crime risk in an area may be sent to an individual's smartphone when they report heightened concerns about the likelihood of victimisation in an area and at a particular time of day. Further to this, real time data can potentially be fed back to local councils and police about the presence of particular neighbourhood problems. This removes many of the existing challenges of traditional fear reduction programs that are typically administered to individuals well after the fact (after experiencing a fearful episode related to crime), or to individuals who have never felt worried about crime in the case of tertiary-level interventions (Renauer 2007).

Physiological monitoring of responses to disorder images. In addition to using smartphone technology to better capture fear of crime and disorder perceptions in the local environment, researchers have also begun to develop and test other sophisticated tools to identify how individual's scan their environments for cues or signs of disorder. This is particularly important, given that existing measures of disorder/incivility have been found to vary across environments and within cultures. That is, what may be perceived as disorder in one group of individuals, may not be considered disorder by another group of individuals. At present, this work is predominantly experimental, and utilises a mixture of visual methods (images of disorderly and/or threatening environments) and ambulatory monitoring of physiological processes (i.e., skin conductance, heart rate, eye tracking etc.). For example, Guedes et al. (2014) used eye tracking technology to understand how individuals selectively attend to particular images. Using a small sample of 10 undergraduate students, Guedes and her colleagues found that people are more likely to attend to negative images of environments (i.e., graffiti, broken windows) than positive and more neutral images of environments. This confirms some of the earlier aforementioned ideas raised by scholars investigating the signals crime perspective, in that individuals' perceptions of crime risk are directly influenced by active signals or cues of out of character behaviour that disrupts the appearance of normalcy in an area.

Virtual auditing of cues of neighbourhood disorder and community health. Finally, other contemporary research has attempted to audit neighbourhood disorder using publicly available images from mapping programs such as Google Street View. Rundle et al. (2011) tested the feasibility of this approach for auditing neighbourhood environmental characteristics such as disorder. They produced concordance rates comparing field audits to data collected from Google Street View for a range of neighbourhood characteristics, including: aesthetics, physical disorder, pedestrian safety, motorized traffic and parking, infrastructure for active travel, sidewalk amenities, and social and commercial activity. Rundle et al. (2011) found high levels of concordance between the measurement of these neighbourhood characteristics between both auditing approaches (about 80% concordance). Interestingly, some neighbourhood characteristics had higher concordance rates between approaches, including pedestrian safety, motorized traffic and parking, and infrastructure for active travel. In contrast, assessments of physical disorder in neighbourhoods produced lower concordance rates between approaches. Rundle et al. (2011) concluded that Google Street View could be a useful neighbourhood auditing tool, given the reasonable concordance rates and the cost effectiveness of this auditing approach.

Similarly, Clarke et al. (2010) concluded that virtual auditing methods using Google Street View can provide reliable indicators of neighbourhood characteristics such as recreational facilities, the local food environment and general land use in a study of Chicago neighbourhoods. However, Clarke et al. (2010) cautions scholars on relying on virtual auditing methods for more fine-grained assessments of neighbourhoods. In the context of assessments of neighbourhood disorder, it is difficult to examine social disorder through the use of static images when adopting virtual approaches such as Google Street View. Nonetheless, virtual audits may allow scholars to detect disorder problems with ease and reduce the costs associated with collecting data on neighbourhood characteristics through objective assessments.

7.7 Concluding Remarks and Future Directions

At the beginning of this chapter we described how fear of crime and disorderly environments may impact upon an individual's quality of life and physical well-being, as well as the broader implications that fear of crime may have on the functioning of society. This was followed by a discussion of the common methods used to evaluate fear of crime and perceptions of disorder in neighbourhoods and public spaces. Later, we described various correlates related to fear of crime, including individual-level variables, neighbourhood-level characteristics, and social characteristics. Moreover, we discussed how these common predictors of fear of crime could be better converged using contemporary social-psychological models that consider the interactions between vulnerability/risk perceptions, perceptions of social and physical environment, and worry about crime.

We concluded this chapter by discussing some new developments in the study of fear of crime, disorder, and quality of life. In particular, we described a number of studies using innovative technological methods (i.e., smartphones, physiological monitoring, and virtual street auditing) to understand the processes behind fear of crime, and to better contextualise and situate fear of crime and subjective perceptions of neighbourhood disorder.

There are a number of possibilities for future research examining the connections between fear of crime, neighbourhood disorder and quality of life. In particular, one future avenue for research may involve the triangulation of different data sources on disorder and fear of crime. At present, few have attempted to consolidate objective and subjective ratings of neighbourhood disorder into single statistical models. This may allow researchers to better test for differences in objective (or actual) levels of disorder in neighbourhoods versus subjective (self-reports) of disorderly neighbourhoods. For example, combining street auditing methods, and local council or law enforcement data (i.e., like fix my street data), with real time data collection on subjective perceptions of disorder across individual's routine activities may provide a more ecologically valid assessment of the prevalence of neighbourhood disorder and its relationship to other social problems such as fear of crime.

Furthermore, cross-cultural differences in subjective perceptions of neighbourhood disorder need to be better acknowledged and investigated further by researchers. Currently, most measures of subjective neighbourhood disorder are adopted from large scale surveys in the United States and United Kingdom, with some of these measures not necessarily being applicable to other countries and environments. For example, in rural Australia, incivilities such as rubbish and litter are less likely to be encountered on a regular basis, in comparison to metropolitan areas, where population density is higher, and therefore the likelihood of encountering rubbish litter in city streets is higher. However, individuals living in rural environments may be more sensitive to social incivilities, given that rural dwellers place more value on relationships and support networks as part of their everyday lives, in comparison to urban dwellers (Reisig and Cancino 2004). Therefore, future work may consider testing perceptions of incivility/neighbourhood disorder at different levels of urbanicity (i.e., urban, rural, and remote), and across different cultures.

Finally, the impacts of fear of crime and neighbourhood disorder on quality of life remain understudied by researchers. Although some research has documented the negative impacts of fear of crime and disorder on quality of life, others have found the opposite effect. That is, healthy levels of fear of crime may have a positive impact on individuals by decreasing their risk of victimisation, through the auctioning of preventative behaviours, such as avoiding crime prone areas (see Melde et al. 2016). There is also a limited amount of research that has attempted to quantify the direct and indirect costs of fear of crime and neighbourhood disorder on individuals and society. Those who have attempted to calculate the tangible and intangible costs of fear of crime on quality of life argue that the inclusion of fear of crime in the overall calculation of costs associated with crime may facilitate more efficient cost-benefit analyses of interventions designed to reduce crime and/or fear of crime (Dolan and Peasgood 2006; Moore and Shepherd 2006).

In sum, the literature on fear of crime, disorder and quality of life is continuing to flourish with new advancements in methods producing exciting new insights into the connections between fear of crime and disorder/incivilities. By better understanding these connections, researchers and policy makers are better positioned to develop more targeted interventions to reduce the occurrence of these problems within communities.

References

Abdullah, A., Marzbali, M. H., Woolley, H., Bahauddin, A., & Maliki, N. Z. (2014). Testing for individual factors for the fear of crime using a multiple indicator-multiple cause model. *European Journal on Criminal Policy and Research, 20*(1), 1–22.

Adams, R. E., & Serpe, R. T. (2000). Social integration, fear of crime, and life satisfaction. *Sociological perspectives, 43*(4), 605–629.

Agnew, R. (1995). Testing the leading crime theories: An alternative strategy focusing on motivational processes. *Journal of research in crime and delinquency, 32*(4), 363–398.

Allen, J. (2006). *Worry about crime in England and Wales: Findings from the 2003/04 and 2004/05 British Crime Survey*. London: Home Office.

Anderson, E. (1990). *Streetwise: Race, class, and change in an urban community*. University of Chicago Press.

Biderman, A. D., Johnson, L., McIntyre, J., & Weir, A. (1967). *Report on a pilot study in the District of Columbia on victimization and attitudes to law enforcement*. US President's commission on Law Enforcement and Administration of Justice, Field Surveys IUS Government Printing Office: Washington DC.

Box, S., Hale, C., & Andrews, G. (1988). Explaining fear of crime. *The British Journal of Criminology, 28*(3), 340–356.

Braungart, M. M., Braungart, R. G., & Hoyer, W. J. (1980). Age, sex, and social factors in fear of crime. *Sociological Focus, 13*(1), 55–66.

Brunton-Smith, I., & Sturgis, P. (2011). Do neighborhoods generate fear of crime? An empirical test using the British Crime Survey. *Criminology, 49*(2), 331–369.

Callanan, V. J., & Teasdale, B. (2009). An exploration of gender differences in measurement of fear of crime. *Feminist Criminology, 4*(4), 359–376.

Chataway, M. L., & Hart, T. C. (2016). (Re)Assessing contemporary "fear of crime" measures within an Australian context. *Journal of Environmental Psychology, 47,* 195–203.

Chataway, M. L., & Hart, T. C. (2018). Crime prevention and reduction programs: How does knowing about community initiatives moderate attitudes towards criminal victimisation? *Australian & New Zealand Journal of Criminology, 51*(2), 239–257.

Chataway, M. L., Hart, T. C., & Bond, C. (2019). The social-psychological process of fearing crime: Developing and testing a new momentary model of victimisation worry. *Australian & New Zealand Journal of Criminology*, 0004865819836153.

Chataway, M. L., Hart, T. C., Coomber, R., & Bond, C. (2017). The geography of crime fear: A pilot study exploring event-based perceptions of risk using mobile technology. *Applied Geography, 86,* 300–307.

Cheshire, L., & Fitzgerald, R. (2015). From private nuisance to criminal behaviour: Neighbour problems and neighbourhood context in an Australian City. *Housing Studies, 30*(1), 100–122.

Clarke, P., Ailshire, J., Melendez, R., Bader, M., & Morenoff, J. (2010). Using Google Earth to conduct a neighborhood audit: Reliability of a virtual audit instrument. *Health & Place, 16*(6), 1224–1229.

Clemente, F., & Kleiman, M. B. (1977). Fear of crime in the United States: A multivariate analysis. *Social Forces, 56*(2), 519–531.

Cops, D., & Pleysier, S. (2010). 'Doing gender' in fear of crime: The impact of gender identity on reported levels of fear of crime in adolescents and young adults. *The British Journal of Criminology, 51*(1), 58–74.

Corcoran, J., Zahnow, R., Wickes, R., & Hipp, J. (2018). Neighbourhood land use features, collective efficacy and local civic actions. *Urban Studies, 55*(11), 2372–2390.

Covington, J., & Taylor, R. B. (1991). Fear of crime in urban residential neighborhoods: Implications of between-and within-neighborhood sources for current models. *The Sociological Quarterly, 32*(2), 231–249.

Crawford, A., Jones, T., Woodhouse, T., & Young, J. (1990). *The second Islington crime survey*. London: Middlesex Polytechnic Centre for Criminology.

Dolan, P., & Peasgood, T. (2006). Estimating the economic and social costs of the fear of crime. *British Journal of Criminology, 47*(1), 121–132.

Ennis, P. H. (1967). *Criminal victimization in the United States: A report of a national survey* (No. 2). Chicago: National Opinion Research Center, University of Chicago.

Farrall, S., Bannister, J., Ditton, J., & Gilchrist, E. (1997). Questioning the measurement of the 'fear of crime': Findings from a major methodological study. *The British Journal of Criminology, 37*(4), 658–679.

Farrall, S., & Gadd, D. (2004). Research note: The frequency of the fear of crime. *British Journal of Criminology, 44*(1), 127–132.

Farrall, S. D., Jackson, J., & Gray, E. (2009). *Social order and the fear of crime in contemporary times*. Oxford: Oxford University Press.

Ferguson, K. M., & Mindel, C. H. (2007). Modeling fear of crime in Dallas neighborhoods: A test of social capital theory. *Crime & Delinquency, 53*(2), 322–349.

Ferraro, K. F. (1995). *Fear of crime: Interpreting victimization risk*. SUNY Press.

Fisher, B. S., & Nasar, J. L. (1992). Fear of crime in relation to three exterior site features: Prospect, refuge, and escape. *Environment and Behavior, 24*(1), 35–65.

Fox, K. A., Nobles, M. R., & Piquero, A. R. (2009). Gender, crime victimization and fear of crime. *Security Journal, 22*(1), 24–39.

Franklin, T. W., Franklin, C. A., & Fearn, N. E. (2008). A multilevel analysis of the vulnerability, disorder, and social integration models of fear of crime. *Social Justice Research, 21*(2), 204–227.

Gabriel, U., & Greve, W. (2003). The psychology of fear of crime. Conceptual and methodological perspectives. *British Journal of Criminology, 43*(3), 600–614.

Gainey, R., Alper, M., & Chappell, A. T. (2011). Fear of crime revisited: Examining the direct and indirect effects of disorder, risk perception, and social capital. *American Journal of Criminal Justice, 36*(2), 120–137.

Garofalo, J. (1981). The fear of crime: Causes and consequences. *Journal of Criminal Law and Criminology, 72,* 839.

Garofalo, J., & Laub, J. (1978). The fear of crime: Broadening our perspective. *Victimology, 3*(3–4), 242–253.

Gazzaniga, M., Ivry, R. B., & Mangun, G. R. (2011). *Cognitive neuroscience: The biology of mind* (3rd ed.). W.W. Norton Company: USA.

Gibson, C. L., Zhao, J., Lovrich, N. P., & Gaffney, M. J. (2002). Social integration, individual perceptions of collective efficacy, and fear of crime in three cities. *Justice Quarterly, 19*(3), 537–564.

Gray, E., Jackson, J., & Farrall, S. (2008). Reassessing the fear of crime. *European Journal of Criminology, 5*(3), 363–380.

Gromet, D. M., & Pronin, E. (2009). What were you worried about? Actors' concerns about revealing fears and insecurities relative to observers' reactions. *Self and Identity, 8*(4), 342–364.

Grubesic, T. H., Wallace, D., Chamberlain, A. W., & Nelson, J. R. (2018). Using unmanned aerial systems (UAS) for remotely sensing physical disorder in neighborhoods. *Landscape and Urban Planning, 169,* 148–159.

Guedes, I., Fernandes, P., & Cardoso, C. (2014). Studying the contextual cues associated with fear of crime through eye tracking techniques. In *ET4S@ GIScience* (pp. 42–46).

Hale, C. (1996). Fear of crime: A review of the literature. *International Review of Victimology, 4* (2), 79–150.

Hanslmaier, M. (2013). Crime, fear and subjective well-being: How victimization and street crime affect fear and life satisfaction. *European Journal of Criminology, 10*(5), 515–533.

Hart, T. C., & Lersch, K. M. (2015). *Space, time, and crime*. Carolina Academic Press.

Herbert, D. T. (1993). Neighbourhood incivilities and the study of crime in place. *Area, 25*(1), 45–54.

Hollway, W., & Jefferson, T. (1997). The risk society in an age of anxiety: Situating fear of crime. *British Journal of Sociology*, 255–266.

Hunter, A. (1978). Symbols of incivility: Social disorder and fear of crime in urban neighborhoods. In *Annual meeting of the american criminological society, Dallas*.
Innes, M. (2004). Signal crimes and signal disorders: Notes on deviance as communicative action 1. *The British Journal of Sociology, 55*(3), 335–355.
Jackson, J. (2004). Experience and expression: Social and cultural significance in the fear of crime. *British Journal of Criminology, 44*(6), 946–966.
Jackson, J. (2005). Validating new measures of the fear of crime. *International Journal of Social Research Methodology, 8*(4), 297–315.
Jackson, J. (2009). A psychological perspective on vulnerability in the fear of crime. *Psychology, Crime & Law, 15*(4), 365–390.
Jackson, J. (2015). Cognitive closure and risk sensitivity in the fear of crime. *Legal and Criminological Psychology, 20*(2), 222–240.
Keane, C. (1998). Evaluating the influence of fear of crime as an environmental mobility restrictor on women's routine activities. *Environment and Behavior, 30*(1), 60–74.
Killias, M. (1990). Vulnerability: Towards a better understanding of a key variable in the genesis of fear of crime. *Violence and Victims, 5*(2), 97–108.
LaGrange, R. L., & Ferraro, K. F. (1989). Assessing age and gender differences in perceived risk and fear of crime. *Criminology, 27*(4), 697–720.
LaGrange, R. L., Ferraro, K. F., & Supancic, M. (1992). Perceived risk and fear of crime: Role of social and physical incivilities. *Journal of Research in Crime and Delinquency, 29*(3), 311–334.
Lane, J., & Meeker, J. W. (2000). Subcultural diversity and the fear of crime and gangs. *Crime & Delinquency, 46*(4), 497–521.
Last, P., & Jackson, S. (1988). *The Bristol fear and risk of crime project: A preliminary report on fear of crime*. Avon and Somerset Constabulary.
Lee, G. R. (1983). Social integration and fear of crime among older persons. *Journal of Gerontology, 38*(6), 745–750.
Lee, M. (2007). *Inventing fear of crime: Criminology and the politics of anxiety*. Cullompton, UK: Willan Publishing.
Lee, M. (2008). The enumeration of anxiety: Power, knowledge and fear of crime. In *Fear of crime* (pp. 44–56). Routledge-Cavendish.
Lee, M. (2013). *Inventing fear of crime*. Willan.
Lee, M., & Mythen, G. (Eds.). (2018). *The Routledge international handbook on fear of crime*. Routledge.
Lewis, D. A., & Salem, G. (1986). *Fear of crime: Incivility and the production of a social problem*. Brunswick, NJ: Transaction.
Liska, A. E., Lawrence, J. J., & Sanchirico, A. (1982). Fear of crime as a social fact. *Social Forces, 60*(3), 760–770.
Liu, J., Messner, S. F., Zhang, L., & Zhuo, Y. (2009). Socio-demographic correlates of fear of crime and the social context of contemporary urban China. *American Journal of Community Psychology, 44*(1–2), 93–108.
Lupton, D., & Tulloch, J. (1999). Theorizing fear of crime: Beyond the rational/irrational opposition. *The British Journal of Sociology, 50*(3), 507–523.
Markowitz, F. E., Bellair, P. E., Liska, A. E., & Liu, J. (2001). Extending social disorganization theory: Modeling the relationships between cohesion, disorder, and fear. *Criminology, 39*(2), 293–319.
Mawby, R. I. (1986). Fear of crime and concern over the crime problem among the elderly. *Journal of Community Psychology, 14*(3), 300–306.
McCrea, R., Shyy, T. K., Western, J., & Stimson, R. J. (2005). Fear of crime in Brisbane: Individual, social and neighbourhood factors in perspective. *Journal of Sociology, 41*(1), 7–27.
McGarrell, E. F., Giacomazzi, A. L., & Thurman, Q. C. (1997). Neighborhood disorder, integration, and the fear of crime. *Justice Quarterly, 14*(3), 479–500.
Melde, C., Berg, M. T., & Esbensen, F. A. (2016). Fear, social interactions, and violence mitigation. *Justice Quarterly, 33*(3), 481–509.

Mesch, G. S. (2000). Perceptions of risk, lifestyle activities, and fear of crime. *Deviant Behavior, 21*(1), 47–62.
Mishra, A., Mishra, H., & Nayakankuppam, D. (2009). The group-contagion effect: The influence of spatial groupings on perceived contagion and preferences. *Psychological Science, 20*(7), 867–870.
Moore, S., & Shepherd, J. P. (2006). The cost of fear: Shadow pricing the intangible costs of crime. *Applied Economics, 38*(3), 293–300.
Ollenburger, J. C. (1981). Criminal victimization and fear of crime. *Research on Aging, 3*(1), 101–118.
Park, R. E., & Burgess, E. W. (1924). *Introduction to the science of sociology* (Vol. 574). Chicago: University of Chicago Press.
Piquero, A. (1999). The validity of incivility measures in public housing. *Justice Quarterly, 16*(4), 793–818.
Putnam, R. (1995). Bowling alone: America's declining social capital. *Journal of Democracy, 6* (1), 64–78.
Rader, N. E., Cossman, J. S., & Porter, J. R. (2012). Fear of crime and vulnerability: Using a national sample of Americans to examiner two competing paradigms. *Journal of Criminal Justice, 40,* 134–141.
Reisig, M. D., & Cancino, J. M. (2004). Incivilities in nonmetropolitan communities: The effects of structural constraints, social conditions, and crime. *Journal of Criminal Justice, 32*(1), 15–29.
Reiss, A. (1967). *Studies in crime and law enforcement in major metropolitan areas.* President's Commission on Law Enforcement and Administration of Justice, Field Surverys III. Washington, DC: US Government Printing Office.
Renauer, B. C. (2007). Reducing fear of crime: Citizen, police, or government responsibility? *Police Quarterly, 10*(1), 41–62.
Ross, C. E., & Jang, S. J. (2000). Neighborhood disorder, fear, and mistrust: The buffering role of social ties with neighbors. *American Journal of Community Psychology, 28*(4), 401–420.
Rountree, P. W., & Land, K. C. (1996). Perceived risk versus fear of crime: Empirical evidence of conceptually distinct reactions in survey data. *Social Forces, 74*(4), 1353–1376.
Rundle, A. G., Bader, M. D., Richards, C. A., Neckerman, K. M., & Teitler, J. O. (2011). Using Google street view to audit neighborhood environments. *American Journal of Preventive Medicine, 40*(1), 94–100.
Sacco, V. F. (1993). Social support and the fear of crime. *Canadian Journal of Criminology, 35,* 187.
Sampson, R. J. (2009). *Shared beginnings, divergent lives.* Harvard University Press.
Sampson, R. J., & Raudenbush, S. W. (1999). Systematic social observation of public spaces: A new look at disorder in urban neighborhoods. *American Journal of Sociology, 105*(3), 603–651.
Sampson, R. J., & Raudenbush, S. W. (2001). *Disorder in urban neighborhoods: Does it lead to crime.* Washington, DC: US Department of Justice, Office of Justice Programs, National Institute of Justice.
Sampson, R. J., & Raudenbush, S. W. (2004). Seeing disorder: Neighborhood stigma and the social construction of "broken windows". *Social Psychology Quarterly, 67*(4), 319–342.
Shaw, C., & McKay, H. (1942). *Juvenile delinquency and urban areas.* Chicago: Chicago University Press.
Shiffman, S. (2009). Ecological momentary assessment (EMA) in studies of substance use. *Psychological Assessment, 21*(4), 486.
Skogan, W. G. (1976). *Sample surveys of the victim of crime.* Cambridge, MA: Ballinger.
Skogan, W. G. (1981). *Issues in the measurement of victimization* (Vol. 200). Washington, DC: US Department of Justice, Bureau of Justice Statistics.
Skogan, W. G. (1990). *Disorder and decline: Crime and the spiral of decay in American Cities.* New York: The Free Press.

Snedker, K. A. (2015). Neighborhood conditions and fear of crime: A reconsideration of sex differences. *Crime & Delinquency, 61*(1), 45–70.
Solymosi, R., Bowers, K., & Fujiyama, T. (2015). Mapping fear of crime as a context-dependent everyday experience that varies in space and time. *Legal and Criminological Psychology, 20* (2), 193–211.
Solymosi, R., Bowers, K. J., & Fujiyama, T. (2017). Crowdsourcing subjective perceptions of neighbourhood disorder: Interpreting bias in open data. *The British Journal of Criminology, 58* (4), 944–967.
Spelman, W. (2004). Optimal targeting of incivility-reduction strategies. *Journal of Quantitative Criminology, 20*(1), 63–88.
Stafford, M., Chandola, T., & Marmot, M. (2007). Association between fear of crime and mental health and physical functioning. *American Journal of Public Health, 97*(11), 2076–2081.
Stanko, E. A. (1995). Women, crime, and fear. *The Annals of the American Academy of Political and Social Science, 539*(1), 46–58.
Taylor, J. (2001). *NCRC Statement at National League of Cities Press Conference*. The State of Cities 2000: Megaforces Shaping the Future of the Nation's Cities. Washington, DC: U.S. Dept. of Housing and Urban Development.
Taylor, R. B., Shumaker, S. A., & Gottfredson, S. D. (1985). Neighborhood-level links between physical features and local sentiments: Deterioration, fear of crime, and confidence. *Journal of Architectural and Planning Research, 2*(4), 261–275.
Thompson, E. E., & Krause, N. (1998). Living alone and neighborhood characteristics as predictors of social support in late life. *The Journals of Gerontology Series B: Psychological Sciences and Social Sciences, 53*(6), 354–364.
Toseland, R. W. (1982). Fear of crime: Who is most vulnerable? *Journal of Criminal Justice, 10* (3), 199–209.
Tsai, L. T., Rantakokko, M., Viljanen, A., Saajanaho, M., Eronen, J., Rantanen, T., et al. (2016). Associations between reasons to go outdoors and objectively-measured walking activity in various life-space areas among older people. *Journal of Aging and Physical Activity, 24*(1), 85–91.
Tseloni, A., & Zarafonitou, C. (2008). Fear of crime and victimization: A multivariate multilevel analysis of competing measurements. *European Journal of Criminology, 5*(4), 387–409.
Van der Wurff, A., Van Staalduinen, L., & Stringer, P. (1989). Fear of crime in residential environments: Testing a social psychological model. *The Journal of Social Psychology, 129*(2), 141–160.
Walker, A., Kershaw, C., & Nicholas, S. (2006). Crime in England and Wales 2005/06. Home office. *Research Methodology, 8*(4), 297–315.
Warner, B. D., & Rountree, P. W. (1997). Local social ties in a community and crime model: Questioning the systemic nature of informal social control. *Social Problems, 44*(4), 520–536.
Warr, M. (1984). Fear of victimization: Why are women and the elderly more afraid? *Social Science Quarterly, 65*(3), 681.
Warr, M. (1990). Dangerous situations: Social context and fear of victimization. *Social Forces, 68* (3), 891–907.
Warr, M. (2000). Fear of crime in the United States: Avenues for research and policy. *Criminal Justice, 4*(4), 451–489.
Weisburd, D., & White, C. (2019). Hot spots of crime are not just hot spots of crime: Examining health outcomes at street segments. *Journal of Contemporary Criminal Justice*, 142–160.
Will, J. A., & McGrath, J. H. (1995). Crime, neighborhood perceptions, and the underclass: The relationship between fear of crime and class position. *Journal of Criminal Justice, 23*(2), 163–176.
Wilson, J. Q., & Kelling, G. L. (1982). Broken windows. *Atlantic Monthly, 249*(3), 29–38.
Windschitl, M. (2002). Framing constructivism in practice as the negotiation of dilemmas: An analysis of the conceptual, pedagogical, cultural, and political challenges facing teachers. *Review of Educational Research, 72*(2), 131–175.

Worrall, J. L. (2006). The discriminant validity of perceptual incivility measures. *Justice Quarterly, 23*(3), 360–383.

Yuan, Y., & McNeeley, S. (2016). Reactions to crime: A multilevel analysis of fear of crime and defensive and participatory behavior. *Journal of Crime and Justice, 39*(4), 455–472.

Chapter 8
Homelessness as a Fusion Policy Problem

Abe Oudshoorn

Many causes of homelessness have been proposed in research, literature, and popular media. These include family conflict, substance use, mental health challenges, lack of education or employment, or even a choice to live rough. These causes largely situate housing loss as an individual experience, perhaps rooted in individual choices or behaviours. However, looking globally, we can see large differentials in rates of homelessness between nations that share many similarities. If homelessness is caused by personal factors, and people globally are more similar than different, then we would predict that rates of homelessness would be fairly stable from nation to nation. However, a quick comparison between the United States, Canada, and Finland, for example, shows three nations with high GDPs per capita having significantly different rates of homelessness. This suggests that homelessness is about much more than individual experiences and is perhaps better explained by differing policy environments.

In this chapter, homelessness will be explored as a fusion policy problem (A Way Home Canada 2019), meaning that many different systems contribute to the existence of this social issue. A policy problem because the structure of social systems creates risk for housing loss and determines supports available in the case of homelessness, and a fusion policy problem due to the many relevant but often disconnected systems such as health care, justice, housing, income support, violence against women/family violence services, and other social services. Particular priority will be given to mental health and substance use as potential causal factors, and the structure of mental health and substance use support systems as relevant illustrations of the relationship between policy and the incidence of homelessness. For consistency of analysis this chapter focuses on the Canadian policy

A. Oudshoorn (✉)
Arthur Labatt Family School of Nursing, Western University,
Room 2304, FIMS & Nursing Building, London, ON N6A 5B9, Canada
e-mail: aoudshoo@gmail.com

K. M. Lersch and J. Chakraborty (eds.), *Geographies of Behavioural Health, Crime, and Disorder*, GeoJournal Library 126,
https://doi.org/10.1007/978-3-030-33467-3_8

environment, but also includes considerations from the United States and Finland for the purpose of comparing and contrasting. While these countries serve as illustrations, the idea of homelessness as a fusion policy problem has international relevance.

8.1 Mental Health Deinstitutionalization and the Rise of Homelessness in Canada

The deinstitutionalization of mental health services and the rise of homelessness in Canada serves as a valuable illustration of fusion policy problems at work and the interconnectedness of health and social problems. There is no doubt that people experiencing homelessness face disproportionate rates of mental health challenges, with surveys frequently indicating rates of mental illness among those experiencing homelessness in and around 1/3 (Nooe and Patterson 2010), and for those chronically homeless, around 90–100% (Krausz et al. 2013). While these data do not speak to the nuance of cause and effect, that is that mental illness can be related to housing loss, but housing loss can also create risk for mental illness (Johnson and Chamberlain 2011), the prevalence is statistically significant. Therefore, it is clear that people living with mental health challenges are disproportionately at risk of homelessness.

The logical question that arises is: How are health services supporting people living with mental health challenges and in what way is the design of services precipitating this risk? The obvious target of concern is the process of mental health deinstitutionalization. Deinstitutionalization is an approach rooted in human rights and the concept that all people have a right to freedom and a right to choices regarding their health care. With mental health care historically rooted in an asylum model, there has been concern going back decades (Everett 1994) that people were being unfairly constrained into often permanent residential care. In Canada, mental health deinstitutionalization dates as far back as the 1960s with a 62% reduction of psychiatric hospital beds in the period of 1964–1979 (Sealy and Whitehead 2004). This deinstitutionalization gained momentum in these time periods as diverse human rights were implemented into policy in Canada. Movements to advance rights for women, people of colour, LGBTQ2S people, and those institutionalized due to a mental illness occurred in parallel.

The timeline of this history is particularly important when then considering the relationship between deinstitutionalization and rates of homelessness in Canada. Deinstitutionalization is often blamed as the sole and/or most relevant policy cause of homelessness (Lamb 1990). However, what is interesting is that there is no evidence to indicate a rise in homelessness through the 1960s and 1970s (Hulchanski 2009) in tandem with this process. Rather, historical documentation points to the mid to late 1980s being the period of rapid increase of homelessness (Hulchanski 2009). While deinstitutionalization is undoubtedly a factor in rates of homelessness (Lamb 1984), it wasn't until the cessation of development of new social housing in Canada in the 1980s that a significant rise in homelessness was observed (Daly 1998). The idea of deinstitutionalization as an abandonment of psychiatric needs has been challenged as a myth (Mossman 1997). As well, homelessness continued to rise across the country well after the end of the deinstitutionalization process (Gaetz et al. 2014) and even while resources for mental health services have again increased (Chow and Priebe 2013). Therefore, this example illustrates how multiple, intersecting policies across sectors precipitate increases in homelessness rather than any single policy or system.

8.2 Defining Relevant Policy Arenas

Consider a hypothetical American family, we will call them the G's, a family of 4 living in rural New York state. While the family is financially stable, with both parents working full-time, Mr. G is at times violent towards both his wife and his two young sons. Mrs. G mentions the abuse she is experiencing one day to the nurse in her primary health care center. The nurse is unsure how to respond and simply states, "If there is anything I can do to help, just let me know." No further action is taken. As the abuse escalates, Mrs. G decides to take the boys to safety, leaving one day while Mr. G is away and travelling to a family shelter in New Jersey. The family's stay in shelter stretches on as Mrs. G avoids going to court for family support out of concern that Mr. G will determine their new location.

In this case, what policy or system is responsible for Mrs. G and her children becoming homeless? There are many:

- If Mr. G had recognized the harmfulness of his behaviours, were there adequate services in place that he could access to learn to be a non-violent partner and father?
- What supports are in place locally for Mrs. G to reach out to early in order to protect herself and her children from violence?
- How could the health system and the nurse in this case have been better prepared to respond to Mrs. G's disclosure in an effective way?
- Can the violence against women sector provide Mrs. G with a better housing option than emergency shelter?
- How could income supports have been provided as an option so that Mrs. G could afford to rent in New Jersey, even temporarily?
- How might the legal system provide for Mrs. G and her children to access support payments while remaining in a location not disclosed to Mr. G?

Therefore, through this case we can see how policies across multiple systems can serve to either increase the risk of homelessness or to prevent housing loss.

8.3 Policies That Cause Homelessness

In this section we will explore evidence in the scholarly literature on particularly common and particularly problematic policies across a variety of systems. While Canadian, American and Finnish policies differ, as it is the total fusion of these diverse policies that sets the foundation for the incidence rate of homelessness, minor international variances are unlikely to have a significant impact on the overall concern presented herein.

Given the relationship between poverty and homelessness (Hanratty 2017), and the overwhelming breadth of policies related to poverty, some boundaries need to be put on the analysis. Conceivably almost any policy domain could be a part of an individual family's story of their journey into homelessness, but this would be pragmatically unwieldy. Therefore, we focus our consideration on six particular policy domains: (1) the health sector, (2) justice system, (3) housing, (4) income supports, (5) violence against women/family violence services, and (6) employment.

8.3.1 Health Sector

A key area of concern that has been identified within the health care sector is discharge planning. Discharge from hospital to homelessness can occur throughout the health care system (Buccieri et al. 2018). It can be the case where an individual has entered into hospital from homelessness and is returning to homelessness, it can also be a case where an individual has lost access to their housing during their hospital stay. The site of care will impact the likelihood of each scenario, with, for example, discharge from homelessness to homelessness occurring frequently in emergency departments, while discharge from housed to homeless is more likely in tertiary mental health services. Of key consideration here is how limitations in discharge planning design can perpetuate or increase the likelihood of housing loss.

Discharge to no fixed address is a controversial practice that has been researched fairly extensively (Buccieri et al. 2018). Of little surprise is that policies that prevent discharge to no fixed address lead to better long-term housing outcomes (Forchuk et al. 2013). However, such policies are not without consequence as the health system then becomes responsible for providing accommodation until housing is obtained and ensuring supports are available to make housing happen. These supports may be provided by hospital staff directly, frequently through social work teams, or may be accessed through partnerships with existing, external community providers (Forchuk et al. 2006). Using existing community providers to house those being discharged is a challenge if, firstly, these providers are already stretched in supporting their own caseloads and may not be open to intake from day-to-day. This means that the hospital is dependent on the availability of staff over whom they have no direct supervision. Secondly, as discussed further below, availability of housing and housing with appropriate supports may be essentially nil, leading to prolonged hospital stays for social versus health reasons. While keeping those with no fixed address in hospital prevents absolute homelessness, the system impact is provision of accommodations in one of the most expensive ways possible. Nuances exist around policies related to discharge to no fixed address in regards to what counts as an address. Most communities consider discharge to shelter as discharge to homelessness (Forchuk et al. 2006), however, for some this meets the criteria of discharge to an address. The same concern relates to temporary, unstable, or unsafe accommodations. Pressures to discharge patients to a permanent address can increase the likelihood of the use of grey market (non-legal, non-conforming) housing options. Therefore, there is a clearly interconnection between housing and health policies as supportive and affordable housing availability supports quality discharge planning.

Loss of one's housing during a hospital stay can also lead to homelessness. This scenario highlights how while homelessness can perceivably happen to anyone, it is most likely to happen to those who experience multiple vulnerabilities such as poverty and unemployment (Mabhala et al. 2016). Firstly, individuals in grey market housing who are not protected by rental contracts are most likely to lose their housing related to a hospital stay. Secondly, those with limited income or whose social assistance income will be decreased in the context of a prolonged hospital stay are also at risk. As tertiary mental health units have a combination of some of the longest lengths of stay (Canadian Institute of Health Information 2005) and high rates of patients with social and financial vulnerabilities (Payne 2006), they are the most likely settings in which hospitalization leads to housing loss. The responsibility for determining the risk of housing loss due to hospitalization lies directly on the health care system as other community supports wouldn't necessarily be aware of the admission. This example demonstrates a clear 'fusion' between income supports, as discussed below, and health services in terms of either increasing or mitigating the risk of homelessness.

8.3.2 *Justice System*

Discharge from a correctional system is another common pathway into homelessness (Fries et al. 2014; Williams et al. 2010). Secondly, punitive versus rehabilitative models of corrections increase risk around root issues of homelessness.

Unlike discharge from hospital, release from a correctional institution can occur on a less clear timeline and is less likely to include follow-up supports (Gaetz and O'Grady 2009). Where discharge from hospital frequently follows a fairly regular care pathway and may be deferred for social reasons, release from corrections can often be relatively sudden related to the outcomes of a court hearing, appeal, bail, reduced sentence. Even in major crimes, with requirements in Canada for a detailed release plan, parole status or earned remission can change quickly and unexpectedly. In this context, the ability to secure housing in advance of release is quite limited unless a release is conditional and an individual is moving to a residential community corrections facility. Although transportation is a requirement on release, there is no requirement for release into housing. Rather, transportation frequently means that individuals are brought directly to an emergency shelter. Conditions of bail or parole can include 'orders to reside', which in the case of those experiencing homelessness or those whose offence means they are to have no contact with the people with whom they formerly resided, are often orders to reside in a particular emergency shelter (Kovacs Group Inc. 2017). While case management teams may be able to arrange for supports upon release, conditional or unconditional, these are in no way guaranteed and case management teams are often too busy with urgent issues to support post-release planning and referrals (Gaetz and O'Grady 2009). This planning is often dependent on the presence and availability of over-stretched community-based organizations such as the John Howard Society or Elizabeth Fry.

A broader discussion than discharge from incarceration is how current corrections models improve or make worse underlying challenges that increase the risk of homelessness. Do individuals with substance use challenges have higher rates of use before or after incarceration? Do individuals with mental health challenges find recovery through rehabilitative services in corrections? Are individuals likely to experience new traumas during incarceration? Does incarceration increase the likelihood of gainful employment? Does incarceration increase social support networks that can mitigate against housing loss? Unfortunately, the answer for each of these questions in both American and Canadian systems is currently overwhelmingly negative (Lambie and Randell 2013). Incarceration increases the likelihood of substance use (Green and Winik 2010), increases mental health challenges (Walker 1983), increases the risk of trauma (Haney 2003), lowers the likelihood of employment (Holzer 2009), and does not increase positive social capital (Rose and Clear 1998). While state and federal institutions play variable lip service to rehabilitation and offer a variety of potentially helpful programs, the overwhelming focus of incarceration is still largely punitive versus rehabilitative. This is not to say that no one enters into substance or mental illness recovery during incarceration and through corrections services, or that no one gains job skills that lead to improved income upon release, but rather that the overall trend is largely negative (Pattillo et al. 2004). Currently, incarceration significantly increases the future risk of homelessness (Metraux et al. 2007).

8.3.3 Housing

The relationship between housing policies and homelessness is perhaps the most intuitive. Where housing is simply too expensive to be affordable by those on assistance, those working part-time or casual hours, or those on minimum wage, communities will see higher rates of homelessness (Hanratty 2017). Two particular elements of housing policy are presented here as significant precipitators of housing loss: Availability of affordable housing, and tenant protections in the context of mental illness and/or substance use.

Across North America, housing costs have consistently outpaced growth in both employment incomes or government supported incomes, particularly in urban areas (Joint Center for Housing Studies of Harvard University 2018). Urban areas are an important focus as in both the U.S. and Canada, populations continue to shift from rural to urban areas (Schaedel et al. 2011). One factor in this upwards pressure is that in developing new housing, whether it is high or low density, the market incentive is to develop in the mid to high end of the market (Searcey 2015). This is because the proportion of fixed land development and construction costs is higher than finishing costs, meaning that spending a bit more to develop higher end housing is an easy way to increase profit margins. Therefore, it increasingly falls to governments to fill in the low end of the housing market. There are no shortage of policy tools to fill this gap, such as housing supplements, renovation credits, grants to developers for new affordable housing, or government-developed housing. However, in stark contrast to other international examples such as Finland (Pleace et al. 2015), communities across North America are simply not providing new affordable housing at a rate consistent with the demand (Gaetz 2010). Where housing is insufficient and unaffordable, there will be homelessness (Moore and Skaburskis 2004).

While insufficient housing supply is one policy factor leading to homelessness, another area of concern is policies that either support or put tenants at risk when they experience a health challenge. For example, a significant proportion of people will experience an episode of mental illness or problematic substance use at some time in their life (Moffitt et al. 2010). As this is a known risk, policy can either heighten or lessen the likelihood that this episode will lead to housing loss. While the incidence of mental health challenges among those experiencing homelessness is high (Nooe and Patterson 2010), leading many to conclude that mental illness causes homelessness, it is notable that the majority of those who encounter a mental illness or addiction do not become homeless. Therefore, mental illness doesn't cause homelessness, rather, problematic policies or insufficient supports means that some who experience health challenges also lose access to housing.

Tenant law and housing rights play a significant role in the relationship between housing, mental health, and homelessness. Where eviction preventions are limited, there is little buffer to support those who encounter a health crisis from losing their housing (Hartman and Robinson 2003). Interrelated to this is that while many jurisdictions have laws to protect individuals from preventable evictions, insufficiency of legal supports can mean that people are ill-informed of these laws or unsupported in accessing their rights under the law. There are assumptions regarding pathways from a mental health challenge to eviction that are worth correcting. Firstly, it is assumed that eviction in the context of mental illness or addiction is always related to tenant behaviours. However, this is incorrect, as some evictions in this context are due to non-payment of rent (Carter 2010). Secondly, it is then often assumed that non-payment of rent should be a simple cause for immediate eviction. However, evidence has shown that most incidences of non-payment of rent can be remediated with the right supports to the satisfaction of tenants and landlords (Kenna et al. 2016). Therefore, it is only in a policy environment that supports easy de-housing of tenants that we see higher relationships between mental health and substance use challenges and homelessness.

Case Example: Vince Nguyen

Vince lives in Portland, Oregon and had worked in a variety of manual labour positions before discovering his true passion, cooking, at the age of 35. However, at the same time he started to notice discomfort in his back and hips. By 2014 things were getting quite difficult for Vince physically and he was diagnosed with ankylosing spondylitis and rheumatoid arthritis. Both are progressive, inflammatory conditions of the bones that can become debilitating, with no known cure. Vince continued to work until standing for even short periods of time became too difficult, and he lost his job in 2015. It was at this time that his mood began to deteriorate.

Unable to afford rent on his downtown, 2-bedroom apartment, he moved into a 1-bedroom just to the northeast of downtown. His new lease was signed with a large property management corporation. Vince did not qualify for TANF and never completed his federal disability benefits application, although at this time he was diagnosed with depression. He began leaving his room rarely and let the last of his relationships deteriorate.

By 2017, Vince had exhausted the last of his savings and in March of that year provided the landlord with only $145 in rent with a promise that he would try to pay more. Eight days into April, Vince received a 3-day notice of eviction. Frustrated that the heat hadn't been working in the unit all winter anyways and not wanting to come face-to-face with a sheriff, Vince simply took his things and went to the Rescue Mission in Burnside. In his second week at the Mission he met with a worker and learned that he could have filed a defence to prevent his eviction based on the lack of heating, but notice had to be given to the landlord prior to moving out. Under Oregon law, because notice wasn't provided in advance, he now has no option to return to the unit or to claim moving expenses, and is responsible to the landlord for the remainder of the rent.

8.3.4 Income Supports

Income supports (colloquially referred to as "welfare") cause homelessness where they are insufficient to meet real housing costs, or insufficient to cover housing costs after basic needs are met.

Income supports are a form of government benefit meant to provide temporary financial relief for those in need. Additionally, income supports can include long-term support for those with a permanent work-limiting disability. In both Canada and the U.S., income support rates tend to vary with higher rates for those with permanent work-limiting disabilities, higher rates for families, higher rates for older adults, and lowest rates for working age single adults. As well, it is worth considering that some jurisdictions have rates that adjust to local cost of living whereas others do not, meaning that high urban housing prices might make rates even less sufficient. Moreover, some jurisdictions have rigorous requirements to access and maintain access such as demonstrated job searching or drug testing (MacDonald et al. 2001). Therefore, several factors will influence sufficiency of income supports such as: family make-up, age, community of residence, cause of need (and the temporary or permanent nature of this cause), requirements to maintain access to income, and policies regarding earning a partial income while receiving assistance.

The province of Ontario, Canada serves as an illustration of how insufficient income support can serve as a pathway into homelessness. Currently, a single adult on social assistance (referred to as 'Ontario Works') receives approximately $750 monthly including tax rebates. Average market rent in large urban areas for a single bedroom apartment is greater than this total income amount, not including funds needed to meet other needs such as food or utilities (eg. One bedroom average market rent in Toronto, ON = $1202; Ottawa, ON = $812; Ministry of Municipal Affairs and Housing 2019). With income supports far below the cost of housing for those temporarily unable to work, they are left with few choices and are at significant risk of homelessness. Housing alternatives such as grey-market housing (non-legal, non-conforming units), tend to be unhealthy and/or unsafe and offer no tenant protections (Hartman and Robinson 2003). As noted above, social housing, often referred to as government housing, involves wait times that stretch into years or even decades (ONPHA 2016). Lastly, newly developed "affordably housing" units are often only required to be at 80% of average market rents (Canada Mortgage and Housing Corporation 2014), meaning that they are still out of reach for single adults on social assistance. Therefore, social assistance rates that are incongruent with real costs of living put all persons accessing social assistance at risk of homelessness.

8.3.5 Violence Against Women/Family Violence Services

For youth and for women in particular, experiences of trauma and family or intimate-partner violence are the most frequently reported contextual factors in pathways into homelessness (Karabanow 2004). Rates of violence and abuse experienced by youth prior to homelessness range from 60 to 70% (Gaetz et al. 2013). Over two thirds of women who are homeless have experienced episodes of interpersonal violence and 61% of women in female-led families in family shelters have experienced intimate-partner violence (Browne and Bassuk 1997). However, it should be emphasized that violence does not cause homelessness. Rather, problematic policies around known social issues create a pathway from experiences of violence to housing loss. As we now detail, this can include school zero-tolerance policies related to youth behaviours, and for women, policies that limit accessing supports such as child welfare policies that deem witnessing family violence as a form of neglect.

Zero tolerance policies in schools are meant to protect youth from experiences of bullying or assault (American Psychological Association Zero Tolerance Task Force 2008). The term 'zero tolerance' means that student perpetrators of bullying and/or violence face automatic sanctions against their actions. This can include automatic expulsion, possibly including school relocation, for students who assault a fellow student, meant to reduce the overall incidence of fighting. However, a critical analysis of such policies uncovers that there are both unintended biases in who is impacted by these policies and the consequences of such policies (Skiba and Knesting 2001). First, research has shown that youth perpetrators of violence in school settings are often victims of violence within the family home (Morrison and D'Incau 1997). Therefore, these policies are more likely to be impacting those who need support related to their own traumas of family violence. Secondly, expulsion, even in the context of relocation, decreases youth access to natural supports in terms of both peer social capital and trusted adults in the form of teachers or administrative staff (Heitzeg 2009). This means that youth who are more likely to have experienced violence in the home, or be experiencing it currently, are then punished by reducing supports for their resilience. We can then see a pathway from family violence to risks for youth homelessness (Giroux 2003).

For women with children who experience intimate partner violence, policies should support them in accessing the help they need to keep both themselves and their children safe. However, child welfare policies at times deem children witnessing violence in the family home as a form of neglect (Nixon et al. 2007). Women who are aware of this policy therefore fear reporting abuse within the home and reaching out for support as they very reasonably fear the risk of child apprehension (same reference as above). Without accessing support, women often stay in abusive relationships until the violence is so severe that they flee for their safety to violence against women shelters. Therefore, poorly considered policies meant to protect children in the context of a violent household can have the unintended consequence of limiting prevention and therefore increasing the risk of housing loss.

8.3.6 Employment

Apart from housing, income support, and child welfare, communities provide an array of other social services. These can be related to employment, child care, senior care, supports for adults with disabilities, supports for refugees and other newcomers, legal aid, or other services to support the well-being of individuals are families. The relationship between policies on employment and experiences of homelessness is illustrated both in terms of ensuring quality of employment and protections in the context of job loss.

Employment precarity can related to homelessness both in the context of being under-employed or in the context of unanticipated job loss (Shinn et al. 2007). Therefore, this points to the potential inadequacy of policies to ensure quality employment or to protect people when employment changes. In regards to quality employment, sufficiency of pay and assurances regarding adequate hours of work help to prevent cases of working poverty whereby those with a job are still unable to meet housing costs. Legislation to support access to unionization has a direct relationship with income sufficiency and worker protections (Uppal 2011). Therefore, jurisdictions that have policies impeding or limiting unionization increase income inequality (Brady et al. 2013; Florida and Mellander 2016) and therefore also the risk of homelessness. Similarly, policy can more or less effectively protect individuals and families in the context of job loss. Where unemployment supports are low, significantly time limited, or conditional, job loss is more likely to lead to homelessness (Steen et al. 2012). In the context of mental health challenges or substance use challenges, employment supports and unionization are interconnected. A union environment is more likely to support workers struggling with health challenges (Brady et al. 2013), and workplace accommodations are related to promoting mental wellness (McDowell and Fossey 2015), thereby cutting off the pathway from a health crisis, to job loss, to housing loss.

8.4 Promising Policies to Prevent Homelessness

So far this chapter has illustrated how intersecting policy domains can serve to increase the risk of individuals and families experiencing homelessness. While the diversity of problematic policies across sectors can be disheartening, conversely it means that the opportunities of effective policy interventions are many. In this section we will explore evidence-based policies across a variety of sectors that can help to prevent or end homelessness. For each, a promising policy approach from the U.S., Canada or Finland will be presented.

8.4.1 Health Sector

In considering promising approaches, we begin by circling back to the opening discussion of mental health deinstitutionalization. An oft-recommended policy that needs to be addressed, as it is frequently presented as a potential improvement, is that of re-institutionalization. That is, there is a consideration that communities need to increase the conditions under which individuals can be involuntarily admitted into mental health care and/or requiring more criteria be met before individuals can be discharged from hospital subsequent to an involuntary admission (Fakhoury and Priebe 2007). While it is fair to assume that increased long-term hospitalization of those experiencing a major mental illness would reduce street homelessness and emergency shelter utilization, this policy would have the ethical limitation of conflicting with human rights (Dennis and Monahan 2013), would be in conflict with research evidence on least-restrictive care, and would have significant financial ramifications due to the significant cost of hospitalization as opposed to housing options in the community. Therefore, it should be noted that increasing mental health related hospitalizations, particularly involuntary admissions, is not recommended as a promising policy approach to reducing homelessness.

Instead, linking the health sector into shared databases and coordinated access is a more promising next step. As noted by Buccieri et al. (2018), where the goal is to discharge people from the hospital into housing, the limitation is availability of or knowledge of housing options. Therefore, policy can serve to bridge this gap. Shared databases is a promising practice being promoted within the homeless-serving sector (Calgary Homeless Foundation 2014), commonly referred to as homelessness management information systems (HMIS). The value of an HMIS is the ability of a large number of small organizations within a region to work more efficiently and effectively to support individuals who access services across multiple organizations (Calgary Homeless Foundation 2014). This can serve to reduce the stress on the client from repeatedly answering the same intake questions, can assist the system as a whole to better identify levels of need and chronicity, and can reduce the costs and challenges faced by small organizations in trying to maintain their own databases. Coordinated access is a second promising practice within the homeless-serving sector (Canadian Alliance to End Homelessness 2018). When done well, coordinated access allows a system to work as a system meaning that there is no wrong door to entry into the system, that those with the highest support needs are provided the highest levels of support, and that availability of services is made clear to all providers (Canadian Alliance to End Homelessness 2018). Within a coordinated access system, organizations use common assessment and intake forms to understand client needs, and through an HMIS can make this information available to other organizations in the system. They can then see what support options are available that align with the client needs, such as whether any Housing First programs are open for intake, supportive housing providers who might be most appropriate for this client, or housing supplements available congruent with the client needs. This allows for the best use of resources by aligning service to need as well as expedites the process of determining availability of services.

Currently, there is a disconnect in most communities between HMIS and coordinated access being implemented in the homeless-serving sector and hospital services (Buccieri et al. 2018). This is understandable as differing data sharing and access legislation between health care organizations and social services can be a barrier to any form of linked client data. However, this limitation is not an absolute barrier and should not be perceived as such. Data sharing is always an option in the context of client consent, so proactive efforts to gain client consent are recommended. Secondly, in the context of planning discharges from hospitals, the direction of data access is those working in the health sector seeing data within an HMIS. This is a simpler process as health information typically has higher criteria for protection than social service information (Ministry of Health and Long-Term Care 2004).

Therefore, integrating health providers involved in hospital discharge planning into HMIS's so that they can participate in coordinated access systems is a promising practice to assist in preventing discharge from hospital to homelessness (Forchuk et al. 2013). This can support health providers to more quickly find services available to clients in the community and more likely make a discharge into affordable housing with the right supports. It will provide for enhanced communication between health and social care providers. It is noted that ethical considerations regarding sharing of data need to be taken seriously within these models. Clear consent needs to always be obtained from individuals whose data is being shared, including to whom and how it will be shared. As well, it is noted that assessment processes that are reduced due to shared data systems are also times for building relationships with clients, so providers should not assume that data in a database is a sufficient basis for moving forward with care if a therapeutic relationship has not been established. However, if these concerns are addressed, the promises of shared data outweigh the risks.

8.4.2 *Justice System*

While discharge planning may be the simpler approach to problematic policies in the justice system, looking to total system reform is more ambitious but more promising. It is a huge barrier to solving homelessness that people who are incarcerated see a decline in their mental health (Walker 1983) and an increase in substance use (Green and Winik 2010). Shifting this fundamental flaw requires more than just better planning and requires a better form of justice as a whole.

Restorative justice is an approach that focuses on rehabilitation of both offenders and the impacted community in the context of a crime (Van Ness and Strong 2014). To date, restorative justice has been implemented in programs internationally, but not as a system-wide approach. This model involves a recognition that the harms of a crime are multi-faceted, effecting relationships, community bonds, potentially causing trauma, and also negatively impacting the offender themselves (Zehr 2015). Therefore, within a restorative justice system, incarceration and punishment involves a focus on healing, reparation, and ultimately reintegration of offenders into communities, and families where appropriate (Oudshoorn 2015). Where current models of justice are punitive, focusing on retribution, restorative justice actually prioritizes offenders taking responsibility for their actions, even empowering them to improve their life circumstances and the circumstances of their community or family (Zehr 2015).

Transformation of justice systems to restorative justice is a promising policy approach to homelessness due to the research evidence regarding this design. Those involved in restorative justice programs have lower rates of recidivism (Bouffard et al. 2017), are more likely to provide restitution for their crime (Van Ness and

Strong 2014), are more likely to engage in substance use recovery (Pettus-Davis et al. 2011), and are more likely to reintegrate into normal daily activities. This demonstrates a profound reversal from the incarceration related trends within the current system noted above.

8.4.3 Housing

The unaffordability of housing internationally may be significantly discouraging as housing costs rising more rapidly than income create a risk for homelessness. However, in spite of the very real concerns, the growth of housing loss related to housing costs is not an inevitability as some jurisdictions are finding promising ways to ensure access to permanent and suitable housing across all income brackets. Finland in particular stands out with three achievements noted in a 2017 analysis of housing across the European Union (EU): "(1) Lowest rate of severe housing deprivation in the EU; (2) Relatively low share of population overburdened by housing costs; (3) Decrease in long-term homelessness" (Housing Europe 2017a, b). In fact, Finland was the only country in all of the EU that saw a reduction in homelessness in 2017.

So, how has Finland ensured access to housing even as private market housing values have increased significantly, in parallel with other European nations? The difference is a consistent and concerted focus on continual development of public housing. Public housing, also referred to as social housing or government housing, is housing provided by a government authority usually requiring proof of low income to access and provided for the purpose of affordability. Affordability can be achieved by subsidizing units or by setting rents according to income (rent-geared-to-income or RGI). Finland has a relatively high proportion of housing stock being public housing at 13% (Housing Europe 2017a), as compared to 4% in Canada (Canada Mortgage and Housing Corporation 2018) and 1.4% in the United States (Dreier and Hulchanski 1993). Including other forms of housing affordability and housing benefits, nearly 30% of Finnish households are receiving some form of subsidization (Housing Europe 2017b).

This current high proportion of public housing in Finland reflects continual investment in development of new public housing. Indeed, proportions of public housing have been much higher in Canada and the United States, with Canada seeing the highest rate of new public housing development in the 1970s, and the U.S. in the 1960s. However, the key differential is that public housing development in Canada and the U.S. has been intermittent at best, with various government administrations increasing or reducing new development, and the Ronald Reagan and George Bush Sr. administrations actually reducing the total supply by demolition of existing units. With the continual growth of populations and the continual rise of housing prices at a pace greater than the rise of income (government or employment income) in years when new public housing development stalls, there is simply growth in waitlists for access to public housing. Because of this, waitlists in communities across Canada and the U.S. now stretch into the years and even decades (ONPHA 2016). Finland, on the other hand, has consistently developed new public housing to match population need, adding for example 8000 units in 2016 (Housing Europe 2017a).

While there are other forms of affordable housing, public/social housing is highlighted herein as the most promising policy approach to preventing and ending homelessness. This is because other forms of affordable housing use affordability criteria set against average market rents. So, for example, a government and non-profit collaboration might develop new 'affordable' housing under an agreement that rents will be no more than 70% of average market rent. However, these rents are still well beyond what is affordable for those with the most limited finances, such as those on social assistance. Alternatively, the RGI models seen in public housing mean that rent is truly affordable for all citizens, and therefore this form of new housing stock is that which is most useful for those exiting homelessness.

8.4.4 Income Supports

Income support is one of the areas where we see the largest differential between U.S. and Canadian policy. In Canada the various provinces and territories have essentially universal income support for all individuals and families with fairly obtainable requirements around demonstrating job searching or readiness. In the U.S. there is greater state-to-state variability and many states where income support is primarily limited to families, veterans, older adults, and those with disabilities rather than being universal. Therefore, potential promising policy reforms will vary significantly across the continent. The recommendation provided herein is for jurisdictions that already provide some form of universal income support for those who are temporarily or permanently unable to work.

Of fundamental importance in the relationship between income support and housing is the adequacy of the income provided (Arapoglou and Gounis 2015). As noted above, where social assistance incomes are below real market rents, people are doomed to either grey market housing or homelessness. Therefore, promising policies align income supports with a true measure of the cost of living. In Canada, it has been proposed that social assistance be aligned with at least one of the measures of poverty, such as the Market Basket Measure (Statistics Canada 2016). This measure is most useful as a benchmark for income support as it reflects local costs of living and adjusts to inflation. This adjustment for inflation is very important because currently social assistance rates are determined as a matter of politics. In this model, each government can decide year-over-year whether to increase, hold, or decrease rates. Rates that don't auto-inflate, i.e. that hold from year to year, are the equivalent of a decrease as cost of living inflates annually. Therefore, auto adjustments of social assistance rates serve to protect individuals and families from housing becoming unaffordable over time. This also benefits landlords who are able to match rent increases to inflation knowing that tenants will have an annual increase in income as well.

Therefore, both setting social assistance rates to at least a minimum real cost of living and ensuring these rates will increase with the cost of living over time is a way to prevent homelessness from outside of the homeless-serving sector.

8.4.5 *Violence Against Women/Family Violence Services*

As noted above, violence and trauma do not inherently lead to homelessness, but rather problematic policies in the lives of those experiencing violence and other forms of marginalization create a risk for housing loss (Baker et al. 2010). Therefore, transforming systems that are not currently optimized to support individuals and families experiencing intersecting forms of discrimination and violence is a promising move towards preventing and ending homelessness. For the purpose of this discussion, it is noted that equity refers to providing the right supports based on differing needs, as opposed to equality which speaks to providing the same supports for all people.

Women experiencing violence and housing instability often experience multiple, intersecting vulnerabilities such as poverty and may experience barriers in support programs such as racial discrimination (Baker et al. 2010). Therefore, transforming services both within the violence against women (VAW) sector and broader health and social services should be focused on equity-oriented care. The EQUIP intervention (EQUIP Health Care 2019), as implemented in British Columbia and Ontario, Canada, provides a promising, evidence-based model (Browne et al. 2015) to evolve services to better support women experiencing violence and trauma.

The EQUIP intervention involves three key dimensions: (1) trauma and violence-informed care; (2) culturally-safe care; and (3) harm reduction. Each of these dimensions is an evidence-based concept that supports more equitable outcomes for otherwise marginalized persons. The intervention involves ten strategies to build organizational capacity in implementing these dimensions. What is notable about this intervention is that although training of staff is a component, this is not the sole element of the intervention. Rather, there is also a significant focus on transforming policies and tailoring services and programs to address inter-related forms of violence. A toolkit is available to support organizations in transforming their work to equity-oriented practice.

Transforming services through an evidence-based approach is a promising approach to prevent homelessness at a structural level for women and families experiencing violence. This is because women leaving violence at times experience further discrimination and traumatization by the services from which they are seeking assistance. Preventing this system failure will help cut off the pathway from domestic violence into homelessness.

8.4.6 Employment

As noted above, employment, and particularly unemployment, have a significant impact on the likelihood of housing loss. Therefore, stability of employment and related protections can prevent the sorts of crises that precipitate homelessness. Also noted above is that unionization is one way to better guarantee worker protections to support individuals through such challenges as a mental illness or addiction. Therefore, one employment sector policy approach to preventing homelessness is allowing for union security agreements.

In brief, union security agreements determine if employees are required to be a member of a union and how union dues are to be collected (Pynes 2004). This allows unions to both ensure that they have sufficient funds for collective bargaining and other functions, and to prevent cases where some employees benefit from the union without paying the costs of its function (Holley et al. 2011). It is noted that in the U.S. context this would not apply to public sector employers as Supreme Court decision of Janus v. AFSCME prevents the requirement of payment of fees by non-union members within the public sector. However, it does challenge the 26 U.S. states that have "right-to-work" legislation the prohibit union security agreements within the private sector as well. Gould and Shierholz (2011) note that these states across comparator employers have lower wages, lower health insurance coverage, and lower pensions. Therefore, replacing right-to-work legislation with the right to union security agreements is a promising policy approach to better protect those in employment from factors leading to housing loss.

8.5 A Future Without Homelessness?

So, what does is mean that homelessness is a fusion policy problem? It means that many public systems contribute as causes of homelessness. This can include discharge into homelessness in the health care system, a justice system that creates harm versus rehabilitation, housing policy that leads to evictions for causes such as experiencing a mental illness, income supports that are insufficient for market rents, child welfare policies that re-victimize women who have experienced domestic violence, and employment sector policies that limit unionization and the related protections for workers. Homelessness often comes at a result of one or more crises experienced by families and therefore limits on protections across public systems increase the risk of this result. The idea that homelessness is caused by mental illness, or family breakdown, or addiction, or injury is too simplistic. Rather, these are causes of homelessness in the case that public systems are insufficiently supportive of those having these experiences. And as these experiences are inevitable globally, supportive policies are needed everywhere.

The good news is that homelessness as a fusion policy problem also means that there are several areas of potential policy intervention. Each potentially problematic system is also a potential system of support. This chapter has outlined a few promising policy directions based on research evidence. This can include common data systems to support hospital discharge to housing, integration of restorative justice models into the corrections system, ongoing development of affordable social housing, income supports that are available and set at a rate congruent with true rental costs, integration of equity oriented models such as EQUIP to reduce the negative impacts of trauma and violence, and guarantees around the ability to unionize to increase worker protections. However, these are only a selection of potential promising policy approaches as there are others. What these approaches illustrate is that best policy practices across a variety of public systems can be protective against housing loss.

We conclude by suggesting that taken in totality, these policy reforms are pathways by which it is possible for societies to actually solve and end homelessness. Indeed, policy reforms are the only way to truly end homelessness.

References

A Way Home Canada. (2019). *Policy*. Retrieved May 27, 2019 from http://awayhome.ca/what-we-do/policy/.

American Psychological Association Zero Tolerance Task Force. (2008). Are zero tolerance policies effective in the schools? An evidentiary review and recommendations. *The American Psychologist, 63*(9), 852.

Arapoglou, V., & Gounis, K. (2015). *Poverty and homelessness in Athens: Governance and the rise of an emergency model of social crisis management*. Hellenic Observatory European Institute, GreeSE Paper No. 90.

Baker, C. K., Billhardt, K. A., Warren, J., Rollins, C., & Glass, N. E. (2010). Domestic violence, housing instability, and homelessness: A review of housing policies and program practices for meeting the needs of survivors. *Aggression and Violent Behavior, 15*(6), 430–439.

Bouffard, J., Cooper, M., & Bergseth, K. (2017). The effectiveness of various restorative justice interventions on recidivism outcomes among juvenile offenders. *Youth Violence and Juvenile Justice, 15*(4), 465–480.

Brady, D., Baker, R. S., & Finnigan, R. (2013). When unionization disappears: State-level unionization and working poverty in the United States. *American Sociological Review, 78*(5), 872–896.

Browne, A., & Bassuk, S. S. (1997). Intimate violence in the lives of homeless and poor housed women: Prevalence and patterns in an ethnically diverse sample. *American Journal of Orthopsychiatry, 67*(2), 261–278.

Browne, A. J., Varcoe, C., Ford-Gilboe, M., & Wathen, C. N. (2015). EQUIP healthcare: An overview of a multi-component intervention to enhance equity-oriented care in primary health care settings. *International Journal for Equity in Health, 14*(1), 152.

Buccieri, K., Oudshoorn, A., Frederick, T., Schiff, R., Abramovich, A., Gaetz, S., et al. (2018). Hospital discharge planning for Canadians experiencing homelessness. *Housing, Care and Support, 22,* 4.

Calgary Homeless Foundation. (2014). *HMIS toolkit*. Retrieved March 2019 from http://calgaryhomeless.com/wp-content/uploads/HMIS-Toolkit-2014.pdf.

Canada Mortgage and Housing Corporation. (2014). *Investment in affordable housing for Ontario (2014 extension) program guidelines*. Retrieved March 2019 from http://www.mah.gov.on.ca/AssetFactory.aspx?did=12338.

Canada Mortgage and Housing Corporation. (2018). *About affordable housing in Canada*. Retrieved April 2019 from https://www.cmhc-schl.gc.ca/en/developing-and-renovating/develop-new-affordable-housing/programs-and-information/about-affordable-housing-in-canada.

Canadian Alliance to End Homelessness. (2018). *What is a coordinated access system?* Retrieved March 2019 from http://caeh.ca/cas/.

Canadian Institute of Health Information. (2005). *Inpatient hospitalizations and average length of stay trends in Canada, 2003–2004 and 2004–2005*. Retrieved March 2019 from https://secure.cihi.ca/free_products/hmdb_analysis_in_brief_e.pdf.

Carter, M. P. (2010). How evictions from subsidized housing routinely violate the rights of persons with mental illness. *Northwestern Journal of Law and Social Policy, 5,* 118.

Chow, W. S., & Priebe, S. (2013). Understanding psychiatric institutionalization: A conceptual review. *BMC Psychiatry, 13*(1), 169.

Daly, G. (1998). Homelessness and the street: Observations from Britain, Canada and the United States. In N. Fyfe (Ed.), *Images of the street: Planning, identity and control in public space* (pp. 111–128).

Dennis, D. L., & Monahan, J. (Eds.). (2013). *Coercion and aggressive community treatment: A new frontier in mental health law*. Springer Science & Business Media.

Dreier, P., & Hulchanski, D. (1993). The role of non-profit housing in Canada and the United States: Some comparisons. *Housing Policy Debate, 4*(1), 43–80.

EQUIP Health Care. (2019). *EQUIP health care: Research to equip health care for equity*. Retrieved April 2019 from https://equiphealthcare.ca/.

Everett, B. (1994). Something is happening: The contemporary consumer and psychiatric survivor movement in historical context. *The Journal of Mind and Behavior*, 55–70.

Fakhoury, W., & Priebe, S. (2007). Deinstitutionalization and reinstitutionalization: Major changes in the provision of mental healthcare. *Psychiatry, 6*(8), 313–316.

Florida, R., & Mellander, C. (2016). The geography of inequality: Difference and determinants of wage and income inequality across US metros. *Regional Studies, 50*(1), 79–92.

Forchuk, C., Godin, M., Hoch, J. S., Kingston-MacClure, S., Jeng, M. S., Puddy, L., et al. (2013). Preventing psychiatric discharge to homelessness. *Canadian Journal of Community Mental Health, 32*(3), 17–28.

Forchuk, C., Russell, G., Kingston-MacClure, S., Turner, K., & Dill, S. (2006). From psychiatric ward to the streets and shelters. *Journal of Psychiatric and Mental Health Nursing, 13*(3), 301–308.

Fries, L., Fedock, G., & Kubiak, S. P. (2014). Role of gender, substance use, and serious mental illness in anticipated postjail homelessness. *Social Work Research, 38*(2), 107–116.

Gaetz, S. (2010). The struggle to end homelessness in Canada: How we created the crisis, and how we can end it. *The Open Health Services and Policy Journal, 3*(21), 21–26.

Gaetz, S., Gulliver, T., & Richter, T. (2014). *The state of homelessness in Canada: 2014*. Toronto: Canadian Observatory on Homelessness Press.

Gaetz, S., & O'Grady, B. (2009). Homelessness, incarceration, and the challenge of effective discharge planning: A Canadian case. In H. J. David, C. Philippa, C. Shirley, H. Stephen, & P. Emily (Eds.) *Finding home: Policy options for addressing homelessness in Canada*. Toronto: Cities Centre, University of Toronto.

Gaetz, S., O'Grady, B., Buccieri, K., Karabanow, J., & Marsolais, A. (2013). *Youth homelessness in Canada: Implications for policy and practice*. Toronto: Canadian Homelessness Research Network Press.

Giroux, H. (2003). Racial injustice and disposable youth in the age of zero tolerance. *International Journal of Qualitative Studies in Education, 16*(4), 553–565.

Gould, E., & Shierholz, H. (2011). The compensation penalty of 'right-to-work' laws. *Economic Policy Institute, Briefing Paper* (p. 299).

Green, D. P., & Winik, D. (2010). Using random judge assignments to estimate the effects of incarceration and probation on recidivism among drug offenders. *Criminology, 48*(2), 357–387.

Haney, C. (2003). *The psychological impact of incarceration: Implications for post-prison adjustment*. Retrieved March 2019 from http://webarchive.urban.org/UploadedPDF/410624_PyschologicalImpact.pdf.

Hanratty, M. (2017). Do local economic conditions affect homelessness? Impact of area housing market factors, unemployment, and poverty on community homeless rates. *Housing Policy Debate, 27*(4), 640–655.

Hartman, C., & Robinson, D. (2003). Evictions: The hidden housing problem. *Housing Policy Debate, 14*(4), 461–501.

Heitzeg, N. A. (2009). Education or Incarceration: Zero tolerance policies and the school to prison pipeline. In *Forum on public policy online* (Vol. 2009, no. 2). Oxford Round Table: Urbana, IL.

Holley, W. H., Jennings, K. M., & Wolters, R. S. (2011). *The labor relations process*. Cengage Learning.

Holzer, H. (2009). Collateral costs: Effects of incarceration on employment and earnings among young workers. *Do prisons make us safer* (pp. 239–265).

Housing Europe. (2017a). *Finland*. Retrieved April 2019 from https://drive.google.com/file/d/0B3Yb8SWGTmE7dl90ZkxqUEx3SFU/view.

Housing Europe. (2017b). *The state of housing in the EU 2017*. Retrieved April 2019 from http://www.housingeurope.eu/file/614/download.

Hulchanski, J. D. (2009). *Homelessness in Canada: Past, present, future*. Cities Centre and Faculty of Social Work, University of Toronto.

Johnson, G., & Chamberlain, C. (2011). Are the homeless mentally ill? *Australian Journal of Social Issues, 46*(1), 29–48.

Joint Center for Housing Studies of Harvard University. (2018). *The state of the nation's housing 2018*. Retrieved March 2019 from https://www.jchs.harvard.edu/sites/default/files/Harvard_JCHS_State_of_the_Nations_Housing_2018.pdf.

Karabanow, J. (2004). *Being young and homeless: Understanding how youth enter and exit street life*. New York: Peter Lang.

Kenna, P., Benjaminsen, L., Busch-Geertsema, V., & Nasarre-Aznar, S. (2016). Pilot project-promoting protection of the right to housing-homelessness prevention in the context of evictions. *European Commission, Directorate-General for Employment, Social Affairs and Inclusion, Luxemburg*.

Kovacs Group Inc. (2017). *Court order to reside pilot project: Final evaluation report*. Retrieved March 2019 from https://www.london.ca/residents/homeless-prevention/Documents/Order%20to%20Reside%20Evaluation%20Report.pdf.

Krausz, R. M., Clarkson, A. F., Strehlau, V., Torchalla, I., Li, K., & Schuetz, C. G. (2013). Mental disorder, service use, and barriers to care among 500 homeless people in 3 different urban settings. *Social Psychiatry and Psychiatric Epidemiology, 48*(8), 1235–1243.

Lamb, H. R. (1984). Deinstitutionalization and the homeless mentally ill. *Psychiatric Services, 35*(9), 899–907.

Lamb, H. R. (1990). Commentary: Will we save the homeless mentally ill? *The American Journal of Psychiatry, 147*(5), 649.

Lambie, I., & Randell, I. (2013). The impact of incarceration on juvenile offenders. *Clinical Psychology Review, 33*(3), 448–459.

Mabhala, M. A., Massey, A., Ellahi, B., & Kingston, P. (2016). Understanding the determinants of homelessness through examining the life stories of homeless people and those who work with them: A qualitative research protocol. *Diversity Equality Health Care, 13*(4), 284–289.

Macdonald, S., Bois, C., Brands, B., Dempsey, D., Erickson, P., Marsh, D., et al. (2001). Drug testing and mandatory treatment for welfare recipients. *International Journal of Drug Policy, 12*(3), 249–257.

McDowell, C., & Fossey, E. (2015). Workplace accommodations for people with mental illness: A scoping review. *Journal of Occupational Rehabilitation, 25*(1), 197–206.

Metraux, S., Roman, C. G., & Cho, R. S. (2007). Incarceration and homelessness. In *National Symposium on Homelessness Research*. US Department of Housing and Urban Development Washington, DC.

Ministry of Health and Long-Term Care. (2004). *Personal health personal health information protection act, 2004: An overview*. Retrieved March 2019 from http://www.health.gov.on.ca/english/providers/project/priv_legislation/overview_leg.pdf.

Ministry of Municipal Affairs and Housing. (2019). *Average market rents in Ontario*. Retrieved March 2019 from http://www.mah.gov.on.ca/Page1117.aspx.

Moffitt, T. E., Caspi, A., Taylor, A., Kokaua, J., Milne, B. J., Polanczyk, G., et al. (2010). How common are common mental disorders? Evidence that lifetime prevalence rates are doubled by prospective versus retrospective ascertainment. *Psychological Medicine, 40*(6), 899–909.

Moore, E., & Skaburskis, A. (2004). Canada's increasing housing affordability burdens. *Housing Studies, 19*(3), 395–413.

Morrison, G. M., & D'Incau, B. (1997). The web of zero-tolerance: Characteristics of students who are recommended for expulsion from school. *Education & Treatment of Children, 20*(3), 316.

Mossman, D. (1997). Deinstitutionalization, homelessness, and the myth of psychiatric abandonment: A structural anthropology perspective. *Social Science and Medicine, 44*(1), 71–83.

Nixon, K. L., Tutty, L. M., Weaver-Dunlop, G., & Walsh, C. A. (2007). Do good intentions beget good policy? A review of child protection policies to address intimate partner violence. *Children and Youth Services Review, 29*(12), 1469–1486.

Nooe, R. M., & Patterson, D. A. (2010). The ecology of homelessness. *Journal of Human Behavior in the Social Environment, 20*(2), 105–152.

ONPHA. (2016). *2016 waiting lists survey report*. Retrieved March 2019 from https://onpha.on.ca/CMDownload.aspx?ContentKey=85812d7f-2d88-4b28-bbb2-9a76990de22d&ContentItemKey=bdeeb1f1-c466-4ffe-a10e-a2b35370e7fe.

Oudshoorn, J. (2015). *Trauma-informed youth justice: A new framework toward a kinder future*. Canadian Scholars' Press.

Pattillo, M., Western, B., & Weiman, D. (Eds.). (2004). *Imprisoning America: The social effects of mass incarceration*. Russell Sage Foundation.

Payne, S. (2006). Mental health, poverty and social exclusion. *Poverty and social exclusion in Britain: The millennium survey* (pp. 285–311).

Pettus-Davis, C., Howard, M. O., Roberts-Lewis, A., & Scheyett, A. M. (2011). Naturally occurring social support in interventions for former prisoners with substance use disorders: Conceptual framework and program model. *Journal of Criminal Justice, 39*(6), 479–488.

Pleace, N., Culhane, D., Granfelt, R., & Knutagård, M. (2015). *The Finnish homelessness strategy–an international review*. Retrieved March 2019 from http://julkaisut.valtioneuvosto.fi/handle/10138/153258.

Pynes, J. (2004). *Human resources management for public and nonprofit organizations* (2nd ed.). Hoboken, NJ: Wiley.

Rose, D. R., & Clear, T. R. (1998). Incarceration, social capital, and crime: Implications for social disorganization theory. *Criminology, 36*(3), 441–480.

Schaedel, R. P., Hardoy, J. E., & Scott-Kinzer, N. (2011). *Urbanization in the Americas from its beginning to the present*. Chicago, IL: Aldine Publishing Company.

Sealy, P., & Whitehead, P. C. (2004). Forty years of deinstitutionalization of psychiatric services in Canada: An empirical assessment. *The Canadian Journal of Psychiatry, 49*(4), 249–257.

Searcey, D. (2015). *In tepid housing market, builders cater to desires of well-off*. Retrieved March 2019 from https://www.nytimes.com/2015/02/25/business/economy/high-end-home-buyers-call-the-tune-in-a-cautious-market.html.

Shinn, M., Gottlieb, J., Wett, J. L., Bahl, A., Cohen, A., & Baron Ellis, D. (2007). Predictors of homelessness among older adults in New York City: Disability, economic, human and social capital and stressful events. *Journal of Health Psychology, 12*(5), 696–708.

Skiba, R. J., & Knesting, K. (2001). Zero tolerance, zero evidence: An analysis of school disciplinary practice. *New Directions for Youth Development, 2001*(92), 17–43.

Statistics Canada. (2016). *Market basket measure (MBM)*. Retrieved April 2019 from https://www12.statcan.gc.ca/nhs-enm/2011/ref/dict/pop165-eng.cfm.

Steen, A., Mackenzie, D., & McCormack, D. (2012). *Homelessness and unemployment: Understanding the connection and breaking the cycle*. Hawthorn: Swinburne Institute for Social Research.

Uppal, S. (2011). Unionization 2011. *Perspectives on Labour and Income, 23*(4), 3.

Van Ness, D. W., & Strong, K. H. (2014). *Restoring justice: An introduction to restorative justice*. Routledge.

Walker, N. (1983). Side-effects of incarceration. *British Journal of Criminology, 23*(1), 61–71.

Williams, B. A., McGuire, J., Lindsay, R. G., Baillargeon, J., Cenzer, I. S., Lee, S. J., et al. (2010). Coming home: Health status and homelessness risk of older pre-release prisoners. *Journal of General Internal Medicine, 25*(10), 1038–1044.

Zehr, H. (2015). *The little book of restorative justice: Revised and updated*. Simon and Schuster.

Chapter 9
Environmental Justice in the US and Beyond: Frameworks, Evidence, and Social Action

Shawna Nadybal, Sara Grineski, Timothy Collins, Alyssa Castor, Aaron Flores, Angel Griego, Casey Mullen and Ricardo Rubio

9.1 Introduction

Our definition of the environment has greatly expanded through time. No longer simply understood as abstract ecosystems or impersonal terrains, the environment has come to represent the quality of the areas in which we live, grow, and define ourselves as human beings. In this sense, the environment is better exemplified by terms such as "home," or "community;" displaying the intimate relationship between the environment and every resident of this planet. But what happens when the environment, this home that we all collectively share, is experienced inequitably by marginalized social groups? As countless studies have shown, environmental risks and benefits are not distributed equally; some of the world's most vulnerable social groups experience disproportionate exposure to environmental hazards while simultaneously lacking the political and economic tools necessary to restructure

---

Alyssa Castor, Aaron Flores, Angel Griego, Casey Mullen, and Ricardo Rubio equally contributed to this chapter.

S. Nadybal · T. Collins (✉) · A. Flores
Department of Geography, Center for Natural and Technological Hazards at the University of Utah, Salt Lake City, USA
e-mail: tim.collins@geog.utah.edu

S. Nadybal
e-mail: shawnanadybal@gmail.com

A. Flores
e-mail: aaron.b.flores@utah.edu

S. Grineski · A. Griego · C. Mullen · R. Rubio
Department of Sociology, Center for Natural and Technological Hazards at the University of Utah, Salt Lake City, USA
e-mail: sara.grineski@soc.utah.edu

K. M. Lersch and J. Chakraborty (eds.), *Geographies of Behavioural Health, Crime, and Disorder*, GeoJournal Library 126,
https://doi.org/10.1007/978-3-030-33467-3_9

their experiences. This means that, despite the fact we each relate to the environment in very personal ways, the nature of that relation is dependent on the privileges and oppressions we experience as members of our respective societies. Quite simply, some disproportionately enjoy the benefits of the environment, while others are unequally exposed to risks.

Existing as both a body of research and a political movement, environmental justice (EJ) has sought to amplify the voices and experiences of environmentally-oppressed social groups and incite meaningful change for them; change that will improve their circumstances and allow them to reach their highest potential as human beings (Bryant 1995). It is clear that the field of EJ does not simply exist to expand scientific knowledge, but to fundamentally rectify the injustices present in contemporary societies. As such, EJ is a work of great magnitude and importance to our world today. The purpose of this chapter is to provide an integrated discussion of theoretical and conceptual issues of EJ, its substantive concerns, global perspectives on EJ, Green Crime as a new derivative of EJ, and social action to promote EJ.

9.2 Theoretical and Conceptual Issues

9.2.1 Definitions of Environmental Justice

While multiple definitions of EJ exist, Bryant (1995, p. 6) defines it as "cultural norms and values, rules, regulations, behaviors, policies, and decisions to support sustainable communities where people can interact with confidence that the environment is safe, nurturing, and productive. EJ is served when people can realize their highest potential." This definition encompasses the core of EJ: all communities, regardless of their demographics, should receive equal treatment and be able to participate in environmental-decision making practices. He (1995, p. 6) continues, "EJ is supported by decent paying safe jobs; quality schools and recreation; decent housing and adequate health care; democratic decision-making and personal empowerment; and communities free of violence, drugs and poverty."

A. Griego
e-mail: u1103010@utah.edu

C. Mullen
e-mail: casey.mullen@utah.edu

R. Rubio
e-mail: rrubio737@gmail.com

S. Grineski · T. Collins · A. Castor
Environmental and Sustainability Studies Program, Center for Natural and Technological Hazards at the University of Utah, Salt Lake City, USA
e-mail: alyssa.castor07@gmail.com

While the definition provided by Bryant (1995) is helpful, what EJ means to a particular community is dependent upon its cultural history, associated movements, and specific desires for justice (Schlosberg 2009). Cultural aspects matter because there is variation in the characteristics of the people who are impacted, as well as *how* they have been impacted. Movements are also important to examine, as they show how a community has chosen to deal with environmental issues; specifically, whether they seek federal assistance, work apart from the government through community-based organizing, or engage in a combination of both (Schlosberg 2009). It is also important to evaluate the degree of resistance exhibited by affected communities and to understand the solutions that the community prefers for the EJ issue at hand. In sum, it is crucial that environmental decision-makers (and EJ scholars) who seek to understand and assist in ameliorating community EJ issues consider the characteristics, values, and preferred actions of the community.

9.2.2 Types of Justice

When thinking about EJ, there are three important types of justice that are relevant to communities seeking environmental equity. The first is distributive justice, which is centered on the belief that social benefits and burdens should be distributed equally among varying communities (Bell and Carrick 2017). Distributive injustice, as such, occurs when these benefits and burdens are apportioned unequally along lines of social positioning. In relation to the environment specifically, distributive injustice could be exemplified by a community of color being disproportionately exposed to pollution from local hazardous waste incinerators. The second is form of justice is procedural justice; this is achieved when state/institutional decision-making processes are performed equitably with respect to the interests and values of diverse stakeholders. When processes are inequitably implemented, stakeholder groups differ in their level of participation according to their social positioning. An exemplar of the resulting procedural injustices could be the exclusion of non-English speaking communities in environmental decision-making processes conducted only in English. Intergenerational justice, another form of justice, reflects both distributive and procedural justice. Specifically, intergenerational justice is action enacted across generations to prevent contemporary injustices from replicating themselves in the future (Schlosberg 2009). In the context of EJ, this could be exemplified by a community receiving effective, long-term solutions to regional water pollution, thereby preventing future residents from experiencing those particular environmental burdens.

9.2.3 Environmental Racism

Environmental racism is a specific case of environmental injustice (Pellow 2000). "Environmental racism refers to any environmental policy, practice, or directive that differentially affects or disadvantages (whether intended or unintended) individuals, groups, or communities based on race, [ethnicity,] or color" (Bullard and Johnson 2000, p. 559). Environmental racism occurs in the US due to the entrenched power structure, whereby whites have historically controlled social institutions, enabling ideologies of white privilege and white supremacy to environmentally marginalize particular groups based on racial constructions. White privilege relates to how whites continue to dominate many segments of social life; it is this power that enables them to monopolize opportunities (Pulido 2015). This oppressive reality has been "justified" through white supremacy, or the belief that whites are superior and therefore entitled to complete ownership of all resources (Pulido 2015). The monopolization of the opportunity structure by whites, often in the forms of educational and economic empowerment, results in substantial race-based inequalities (Pulido 2015). As a result, environmental racism becomes the visible outcomes of these dynamics.

9.2.4 Development of Environmental Injustices

Environmental racism and injustices emerge through complex processes that Pellow (2000) relates to linkages between socio-historical process and multi-stakeholder negotiations. Socio-historical processes have shaped environmental injustices (Pellow 2000). In US history, race has served as the most influential factor in environmental injustices. In regard to how and why race operates, historical relations have profoundly influenced how marginalized groups have settled and lived. For example, the experience of slavery for African-Americans ultimately lead to segregation, which affected not only their housing situations, but also their levels of education, economic resources, and social power. While this is only one example, it nonetheless suggests how certain racial groups (particularly whites) have historically benefited from the structural oppression of other demographics (Pellow 2000).

Fights for EJ involve multiple stakeholders with shifting interests and allegiances that do not conform to the traditional one victim-one perpetrator scenario. When thinking of EJ issues, it is easy to assume that targeted communities are monolithic and simply overpowered, but this is rarely the case. Opening a toxic waste facility, for example, typically requires negotiation with stakeholders and members of the affected community (Pellow 2000). Desires within the community may be complex and multifaceted and it is often not possible to effectuate broad-based resistance due the distribution of power both within and beyond the community. Stakeholder interests may also change over time, further complicating decision-making (Pellow 2000).

9.3 Substantive Concerns

Those conceptual underpinnings have been substantiated and further developed through more than 35 years of empirical research on distributive EJ. This section provides an overview of the substantive contributions to knowledge made by distributive EJ research in the US and other world regions, as well as new knowledge of EJ flowing from the emerging field of green criminology.

9.3.1 US Perspectives

9.3.1.1 Race and Ethnicity

The United Church of Christ (UCC 1987) sponsored the first study to identify race as the strongest predictor of location for hazardous and toxic waste facilities in the United States. It established an important relationship between race and toxic pollution—one indicating unequal environmental burdens for communities of color—that has been subsequently found across a multitude of other studies. Soon thereafter, for example, Bullard's (1994) classic work highlighted how racial/ethnic minority communities were disproportionately affected by locally unwanted land uses (LULUs), including energy production facilities, toxic waste facilities, and landfills. In the ensuing decades, other researchers have documented that air pollution, soil pollution, lead poisoning, water contamination, and the location of landfills, toxic and solid waste facilities, and incinerators disproportionately burden African American populations (Ash and Boyce 2018; Brulle and Pellow 2005a, b; Bullard 1993; Bullard and Johnson 2000; Mohai et al. 2009).

African Americans were the initial focus in EJ literature, but the scope has since expanded to document similar discriminatory patterns for Hispanics and Asian Americans (Grineski et al. 2013, 2017). For example, in US census tracts, an increase in the proportion of Hispanic and Asian American residents relative to the proportion of white residents is associated with a significantly higher lifetime cancer risk from hazardous air pollutants (Grineski et al. 2017). Native Americans have been also been of focus in studies documenting their disproportionate exposure to contamination of food and water supplies (Gochfeld and Burger 2011; Harris and Harper 1997, 2011).

9.3.1.2 Socioeconomic Status (SES)

Though race is most important in the US context, socioeconomic status (SES; often measured by income, educational attainment, occupational status, and housing tenure) is also a strong correlate for the distribution of environmental hazards. For example, a statewide study in North Carolina found that increases in household income were associated with lower concentrations of particulate matter less than 2.5 μm in diameter ($PM_{2.5}$), a type of air pollutant which poses well-known risks to human health, at the census tract-scale (Gray et al. 2013). Higher concentrations of $PM_{2.5}$ were also associated with increases in the percent of the population in poverty and percent with less than a high school education (Gray et al. 2013). Noise from road traffic, air traffic, and industry also have documented associations with SES, as researchers have found that census block groups in the contiguous U.S. with higher proportions of renters, impoverished people, unemployed residents, and residents with less than a high school education are disproportionately exposed to noise pollution (Casey et al. 2017). In a national study, researchers found that renter status, lower income and lower education were associated with greater exposure to pollution from Toxics Release Inventory (TRI) facilities (Pais et al. 2014), which include large industrial point sources of pollution. Apart from residential exposure, people of low SES are also more likely to work jobs that may increase their exposure to hazardous chemicals (Evans and Kantrowitz 2002). In Phoenix, Arizona, where extreme heat is a locally relevant hazard, low-income neighborhoods contain less green vegetation, increasing their exposure to extreme surface temperatures and heat stress (Harlan et al. 2006; Jenerette et al. 2007).

9.3.1.3 Gender and Sexual Orientation

While studied less often than race and SES, gender and sexual orientation are also predictive of disproportionate hazard exposure and therefore important to include in the conversation. In terms of gender, single-mother households are overrepresented in US census tracts that are located near industrial facilities; and controlling for other variables including race and SES, tracts with higher percentages of single mother households (relative to other types of family groups) were also exposed to greater concentrations of toxic chemicals (Downey and Hawkins 2008). Census block groups in El Paso county (Texas) with high proportions of female-headed households (with or without children) were found to be more exposed to hazardous air pollutants as compared to census block groups with low proportions of female-headed households (Collins et al. 2011).

Building off this earlier focus on gender, recent EJ research has examined associations between sexual orientation and the degree of hazard exposure. The first study to examine this found that census tracts in the Houston Metropolitan Statistical Area (MSA) with clusters of same-sex partner households were predictive of exposure and cancer risks from hazardous air pollutants (Collins et al. 2017a). A national follow-up study found that same-sex partner enclaves in the US experience disproportionately high exposure to hazardous air pollutants, and that the associations were stronger than they were for the proportion black and Hispanic resident variables. The same-sex partner finding is largely driven by the presence of gay male partners, as they were associated with greater residential air pollutant risks than was lesbian partnering (Collins et al. 2017b). This pattern has resulted from the social stigmatization of sexual minorities and their spatial exclusion with other marginalized people and LULUs in inner-city spaces across many US cities (Collins et al. 2017b); this process has been more acute for men as lesbian women have a more dispersed pattern of residence (Spring 2013).

9.3.1.4 Immigrant Status

Though less often examined in EJ literature, immigrant status is an important variable to consider. The foreign-born population is rapidly growing in the US and is projected to reach 42 million by 2025 (Cunningham et al. 2008); this indicates a need to better understand how immigrant populations are affected by environmental hazards. Immigrants tend to reside in urban areas where employment opportunities are abundant, where housing is cheaper, and where public transportation is sufficient (Massey 1985). US counties with large proportions of hazardous waste facilities and Superfund sites are more likely to have high percentages of immigrant populations (Hunter 2006). Superfund sites are designated by the US EPA as needing long-term cleanup of hazardous waste. In El Paso county (Texas), census block groups with the highest proportions of residents who were not born in the US and who were not citizens of the US were found to be disproportionately exposed to carcinogenic air pollution relative to block groups with the lowest proportions of those two variables (Collins et al. 2011). A qualitative interview-based study with local Hispanic householders in Greater Houston, Texas offers potential explanations for why immigrant households have greater exposure than other households. While both immigrant and non-immigrant Hispanic households in the study were constrained economically from accessing less polluted environments, immigrant households were attracted to the sociocultural benefits of living in co-ethnic enclaves, e.g., proximity to work opportunities and family members feeling more comfortable and secure in their communities, which led them to environmentally riskier neighborhoods (Hernandez et al. 2015).

9.3.1.5 Intracategorical Studies

Without dismissing the studies noted above, analyses focused on racial/ethnic differences in hazard exposure have typically used monolithic race and ethnicity variables when assessing environmental inequalities (such as percentage of census tract residents who are Black or Hispanic) (Ard 2015; Chakraborty 2009; Downey and Hawkins 2008). This approach to categorizing race/ethnicity fails to account for complex differences within racial/ethnic groups. A consideration of within-group differences can be achieved through an intracategorical approach, first introduced by McCall (2005) in her influential work on "intersectionality." This method "[focuses] on particular social groups at neglected points of intersection…in order to reveal the complexity of lived experience within such groups" (McCall 2005, p. 1773).

Intracategorical approaches for examining differences within racial/ethnic groups were first introduced to EJ research by Collins et al. (2011). Specifically, they applied an intracategorical lens to study unequal risk to hazardous air pollutants in El Paso, Texas, which identified several risk factors within the Hispanic population (e.g., lack of English proficiency, foreign-birth, age over 65, and low social class). This initial effort led to subsequent intracategorical studies (e.g., Grineski et al. 2013, 2015; Chakraborty et al. 2017), which applied the approach to Latino/a populations in several US cities.

For example, several studies were conducted in Miami due to its large and diverse Hispanic population. An individual-level study found that people of Cuban descent were more likely to reside in Miami neighborhoods disproportionately exposed to traffic pollution than non-Hispanic Whites and members of other Hispanic ancestral groups (i.e., Colombian, Mexican and Puerto Rican) (Chakraborty et al. 2017). The same study also found increased risks for unemployed versus employed Hispanics and foreign-born versus US-born Hispanics. A census tract level study also found that Miami neighborhoods with higher percentages of people of Cuban and Colombian ancestry (relative to non-Hispanic Whites) had higher levels of traffic pollution, but those with high percentages of people of Mexican descent had lower levels (Grineski et al. 2013).

While the majority of intracategorical EJ studies have focused on Hispanic populations, other recent research efforts have expanded this approach to other social groups. Within Asian populations, for example, a national study found intra-ethnic differences in relation to cancer risk from hazardous air pollutants. Specifically, neighborhoods with higher percentages of Chinese, Korean, and South Asians (relative to the percentage of whites) had significantly higher risk. Tracts with higher concentrations of Asians speaking a non-English language (vs. those speaking English) and Asians that are US-born (vs. those that are foreign-born) also had significantly greater risks from hazardous air pollutants (Grineski et al. 2017). On a smaller spatial scale, women of Japanese and Korean ancestry in California had significantly higher exposure to carcinogens linked to breast cancer than white women; this was otherwise masked by considering Asians alone (Quach et al. 2014). Similar results have also been found for Black Americans living in economically-deprived census tracts (Liévanos 2015). These studies reinforce the importance and value of intracategorical perspectives in US EJ studies.

9.3.2 Global Perspectives

In analyzing the influence of these variables on hazard exposure and risk, it is clear that environmental injustices are well documented in the US. This makes sense, as both the EJ movement and research field originated in the United States. However, research has revealed that other world regions exhibit patterns of environmental injustice. Research efforts such as the EJ Atlas, which documents global social conflicts as they exist in relation to the environment, help contextualize the widespread dynamics of environmental injustice (Temper et al. 2015). In addition, the work of other leading EJ researchers can draw attention to the globalized political and economic processes that are often responsible for these situations and their tendency to marginalize the world's most vulnerable populations (Bullard and Lewis 1996; Cutter 1995; Pellow 2007).

In the following section, we discuss specific world regions on an individual basis to clarify their specific dynamics of environmental injustice. We focus on environmental injustices in Europe, Latin America, and Asia. While the still-generating nature of EJ research limits our ability to adequately cover other major world regions such as Africa, the Middle East, and Oceania, we include brief descriptions of well-documented cases. Our review is primarily limited to the English language literature.

9.3.2.1 Europe

Like other developed world regions, efforts towards economic prosperity have coincided with the creation of disproportionate hazard exposure in Europe (Laurent 2011). This is particularly true along lines of SES, which has been examined more often than race in European EJ studies. For example, a study of the European Union in its entirety showed a correlation between lower levels of income and employment (both of which are major indicators for economic marginalization) and higher levels of refinery emissions (Gouldson 2006). A similar study in Hamburg, Germany found that toxic release facilities were disproportionately located within impoverished neighborhoods (Raddatz and Mennis 2013).

Apart from SES, immigrant status has also been associated with exposures in Europe. For example, the Hamburg study also found that the facilities were disproportionately situated in communities with higher immigrant concentrations (Raddatz and Mennis 2013). Similarly, French towns with higher proportions of foreign-born residents were more likely to house hazardous waste facilities than those with larger French-born populations (Laurian 2008). Such patterns were also replicated in Italy, where agricultural migrant workers face serious health risks from toxic pesticides and harsh working conditions (Perrotta 2016). In this sense, there are clear disparities along the lines of immigrant status in Europe.

While studied less often, there are racial/ethnic patterns of inequality in Europe too. Roma communities are perhaps one of the most important examples of this, as their experiences as an ethnic minority in multiple European countries can shed light on the EJ dynamics of the region at large. Several studies have found that landfills or illegal waste dumps are often concentrated in Roma communities, alongside limited access to clean water, and communal green spaces and other important environmental resources (Harper et al. 2009; Steger and Filčák 2008). While these patterns of ethnic and racial discrimination do not always present themselves in other European contexts (see Jones et al. 2009), their widespread presence in Roma communities nonetheless indicates the influence of race/ethnicity in regional environmental injustices.

9.3.2.2 Latin American: The Global South

While still developing, EJ research efforts in Latin America are generally oriented toward the repercussions of economic development. These studies have mainly focused on the urbanization patterns present in the continent and Caribbean, as an estimated 80% of residents now live in urban settings (United Nations 2014). Due to the rapid nature of this demographic shift, it has been difficult for respective governments to prevent the construction of informal shanty towns along urban peripheries (Jiménez 2015). These settlements, generally comprised of socioeconomically-marginalized citizens, tend to be disproportionately affected by natural hazards, industrial pollutants, and lack access to both clean water and effective waste management (Vasquez et al. 2018). In this sense, they experience significant environmental injustices as a result of economic endeavors present in the region.

Similar dynamics have also presented themselves along the US-Mexico border. As the maquiladora (export processing) economic sector has grown, hazardous methods of production have generally been exported to American-owned factories in Mexico (Grineski and Juárez-Carrillo 2012). This has led to disproportionate degrees of pollution and environmental degradation in Mexican territories, though specifically in impoverished areas without stable infrastructure, waste management, and piped water (Grineski and Collins 2010). Because the maquiladora sector offers employment opportunities that are inaccessible in other locations, migrants from more marginal parts of Mexico continue to come to the border region and experience the health repercussions of these environmental injustices (Grineski and Juárez-Carrillo 2012).

Research in Chile has demonstrated major environmental injustices, specifically in relation to its neoliberal political structure, intense urbanization, and geographic susceptibility to natural hazards. For example, the country is home to several moderately-sized cities labeled "sacrifice zones" due to their high levels of industrial pollutants (Vasquez et al. 2018). These areas suffer from high rates of poverty, limited access to clean water, and insufficient public services (Fundacion Terram 2014). Though some efforts are being made to correct these issues by local governments, distributional and procedural environmental injustices persist in Latin America.

9.3.2.3 Asia

Though Asia is also a relatively new region for EJ research, several influential studies in China have uncovered disproportionate exposure to environmental hazards. This is best summarized by the cancer village phenomenon present in mainland regions, where the number of cancer patients in certain territories is abnormally high (Liu 2010). This disparity is thought to be the result of water pollution resulting from economic development and is generally more concentrated in impoverished villages (Liu 2010). Similarly, economically-marginalized residents of Hong Kong have been exposed to higher concentrations of vehicular air pollution than their wealthier counterparts (Fan et al. 2012). These findings suggest that socioeconomic status is an influential variable for environmental inequalities in China.

Residents of South and Southeast Asia also experience patterns of environmental discrimination, with documented cases mainly being associated with resource extraction and utilization. These patterns of injustice are primarily due to the levels of economic marginalization present in these regions, as poverty creates both a dependency on natural resources and a vulnerability to their economic exploitation. In Bangladesh, for example, some subsistence-based Indigenous groups have experienced decreased access to vital resources as a result of the non-Indigenous population's economic ventures, social privileges, and nonobservance of subsistence-based lifestyles (Cha 2006). Similarly, the growth of Thailand's economy and subsequent electricity demands have led to the exportation of power projects to marginalized communities in both Laos and Myanmar (Middleton 2012). While economic disenfranchisement is partially to blame for these disparities, both Laos and Myanmar exhibit serious restrictions to community organization and media freedom that can be important tools of resistance (a reality that has been proven by Thai communities' own success with environmental protest and forced-relocation of energy projects) (Middleton 2012). What this means, then, is that vulnerable Lao and Myanmarese people are bearing the social and environmental costs that come with such endeavors without receiving many benefits. The costs include pollution, increased likelihood of hazard, and decreased access to the natural resources upon which rural communities are dependent.

In discussing EJ research in South Asia, it is important to focus on India specifically due to its identification as one of the major emerging economies of the world. As other examples have indicated, economic development is often associated with the presence of environmental injustices for vulnerable communities. Chakraborty and Basu (2019) found evidence of this in relation to the placement of industrial facilities known as major accident hazard (MAH) units. It was found that socially-disadvantaged communities such as those with high concentrations of people from Scheduled Castes and Scheduled Tribes house higher densities of non-publicly funded MAHs. Additionally, variables representing economic marginalization (e.g. higher urbanization and lower home ownership) were also predictive of MAH density (Chakraborty and Basu 2019). This pattern of environmental injustice was similar to that found in a national level study, which found that districts in India with higher proportions of socioeconomically-marginalized people were more likely to be large generators of hazardous waste (Basu and Chakraborty 2016).

9.3.2.4 Africa, the Middle East and Oceania

Though the EJ literature is not as well developed, it is important to briefly discuss environmental injustices as they exist in Africa, the Middle East, and Oceania; this will allow for a more comprehensive analysis of EJ issues from a global perspective. Beginning first with Africa, most EJ research has been oriented in South Africa due to the repercussions of its apartheid system (Leonard 2018). The institution of apartheid, along with its promotion of systemic racism, led to a situation in which regional mining companies often acted without regulation; corporations were therefore able to influence the construction and application of governmental policies. When apartheid ended, the political influence of mining companies still remained, which led to a decrease in decision-making opportunities for socially marginalized communities and the disproportionate placement of polluting mines in their communities (Leonard 2018). Similar dynamics have presented themselves in the sub-Saharan countries of Nigeria, Ghana, and Uganda. Because people in these countries typically lack technical skills and access to capital as a result of marginalization, they have essentially been forced to rely on multinational enterprises (MNEs) to utilize and export their natural resources (Aldinger 2013). These industries, often located in the poorest, most isolated communities in the country, include energy projects that are responsible for major water and air pollution, denial of access to traditional lands, and deforestation (Aldinger 2013).

The Middle East also houses environmental injustices, though these have only been briefly examined when compared to other world regions like the Global North and the Global South. Regardless, the literature that does exist generally indicates major disparities based on lines of race/ethnicity and economy status in Israel. For example, a study found that green spaces in mixed-race cities (e.g. where both Arab and Israelis inhabit the city rather than in ethnic enclaves) are substantially less accessible to the Arab population and economically-marginalized demographics (Omer and Or 2005). Similarly, Shmueli found that Arab populations experience the hazards of industrial parks located within neighboring Jewish communities while gaining none of the revenues generated by the facilities (2008). This is not surprising when coupled with other contributions to the literature, which have indicated that Arab-identifying residents of Israel receive poorer forms of waste management than their Israeli counterparts (Tal 2002), and also earn less income (Omer and Or 2005). Similar patterns of environmental injustice are also present in Iraq and Afghanistan. For example, US military efforts that have frequented these areas often burn their solid waste in open pits near civilian populations, leading to their exposure to hazardous emissions (Bonds 2016). This is essentially exclusionary environmental decision-making, which, as discussed, is a fundamental basis for environmental injustice.

Most of the EJ literature for Oceania is oriented toward Australia; specifically, within the country's Indigenous communities. This can be predominately attributed to Australia's colonial past, which has led to the racial and economic marginalization of Native peoples on a systemic basis. The heavy presence of asbestos mining in Australia's history is a strong testament to this dynamic. Due to a lack of economic power and environmental decision-making opportunities, Indigenous communities often housed asbestos mines in their communities, and were even specifically recruited to work in the mines (Webster 2005; Maloney 2014). This is a particularly pernicious environmental injustice due to asbestos' linkages with mesothelioma, a deadly form of lung cancer. The first Australian national study of industrial air pollution found that communities with greater proportions of Indigenous and economically-marginalized residents contain larger numbers of polluting sites and emit higher volumes of pollutants (Chakraborty and Green 2014). Native communities in Australia have also had to fight vigilantly to prevent the disproportionate placement of nuclear facilities in their communities (Maloney 2014); as such, the patterns of environmental injustice in Australia are quite clear.

In discussing Oceania, it is important to include environmental injustices that occur in the Carteret Islands, Cook Islands, Kiribati, Tokelau, the Federated States of Micronesia, and other oceanic regions as a result of climate change and sea level rise (Brindal 2007). It is estimated that in one hundred years' time, many of these nations will be inundated with ocean water and rendered uninhabitable to the Indigenous and socioeconomically marginalized communities that reside there. Despite the fact that regions such as these contribute the least to global emissions and rising sea levels, they disproportionately experience the effects of climate change and its harmful repercussions (Brindal 2007).

9.3.3 Green Criminology

As reviewed in the previous section, environmental injustices transcend international boundaries and influence various social groups around the world. This raises a question about what broader dynamics are at play that encourage the development of socioenvironmental disparities. Green criminology, which is a blend of criminology and EJ research, seeks to answer this question (Lynch and Stretesky 2014). Green crime is defined as actions or behaviors from corporations and individuals that have the potential to cause harm to the environment, humans, and non-human species (Lynch and Barrett 2018; Stretesky et al. 2013; Lynch and Stretesky 2013). Green criminology is an emerging field that studies green crime with a particular focus on understanding the economic drivers of environmental injustices. While this review focuses on negative impacts on humans (particularly those in disadvantaged communities), it is important to note that there are subfields within green criminology that analyze the negative impacts of industrial production on ecological systems, rates of extinction, and animal rights.

An important factor in green criminology that has delayed the field's progression has been the criminological tradition of narrowly defining crimes from an exclusively legal standpoint (Lynch and Barrett 2018; Lynch 1990). Crimes committed by corporations are often considered legal even if they significantly degrade the environment. Green criminology, in contrast, defines crime as the point at which the environment and its inhabitants are negatively affected by industrial activities

(Lynch and Barrett 2018). This definition is important when considering the influence that powerful corporations have on constructing the extent of legality, as they often encourage the separation of crime from the environment so as to absolve themselves of responsibility for their contributions to environmental degradation.

This has major implications to the environment, especially for marginalized communities who, as EJ literature teaches us, often bear the burdens of these crimes. Lynch and Barrett (2018) highlight this in citing evidence that petrochemical refineries in Black, Hispanic and low SES communities receive lesser punishments for environmental violations. Their privileged legal treatment allows refineries to focus their production processes exclusively on maximizing profit, despite the serious health ailments they cause in surrounding communities (Mohai et al. 2009). By fusing EJ and criminology, green criminology facilitates understanding of how minority populations' health and wellbeing are disproportionately impacted when environmental regulations are disregarded.

Green criminology also sheds light on how capitalism negatively influences corporate interests and industrial production in relation to the environment. The primary focus of capitalism is expansion and production of goods for accumulation. When accumulation of capital is at the epicenter of what markets deem necessary for success, green crime abounds. The globalization of capitalistic trade creates demands for profitability and productivity across world regions, and global capitalism's emphasis on profitability creates socioenvironmental predicaments (Lynch and Stretesky 2013). Green criminology places the reduction and elimination of environmental harm above all else as it seeks to challenge the structures from which many green crimes and environmental injustices derive.

For green criminologists, heavy exposure to toxic substances such as lead, mercury, and cadmium reflects a notable form of green crime; this is due to the association of these substances with severe infirmities such as loss of brain matter, inhibition and disruption of cognitive development, and gliosis (i.e. scarring of the brain) (Lynch and Stretesky 2013). The Love Canal landfill disaster, widely considered one of the first documented cases of green crime, is an important example of this green criminology emphasis (Ruggiero and South 2010). In the 1940s, thousands of barrels of toxic chemical waste were dumped into an abandoned canal by the Hooker Chemical company in Niagara Falls, New York. The site was eventually covered in the 1950s, where it was then purchased by the Niagara Falls Board of Education. This occurred without full knowledge of the area's chemical history, meaning both homes and a school were built there, despite the risk this posed to residents. It was only when heavy rains brought these toxic chemicals to the surface that residents became aware of the environmental degradation of their community (Ruggiero and South 2010). The understanding of such cases paves the way for environmental justice advocates to better recognize green crime and develop approaches to support affected communities.

In discussing inequitable chemical exposure, it is instructive to focus on lead specifically. Excessive lead exposure is associated with higher rates of aggravated assault (Lersch and Hart 2014); as such, lead has a known capacity to influence behavior within exposed communities. This is of particular importance for racial and ethnic minorities, since they are disproportionately exposed (Stretesky 2003) and thus more susceptible to lead-induced behavioral changes (e.g., engagement in violent crime). Behavioral changes flowing from their unjust lead exposures may result in their being criminalized (i.e., stigmatized as hyper-violent), further reinforcing their social, economic, and environmental marginalization. Such a dynamic demonstrates how corporate disregard for the environment can translate into the deepening of inequitable social structures for racial and ethnic minorities. This example illustrates the complex effects that environmental injustice can have on communities.

Green criminology research points toward the influence of capitalism in shaping behavior in the corporate realm, which negatively impacts the health and wellness of racial/ethnic minority and lower SES populations. Without laws to govern corporate interests, organized green crime will continue to degrade both the health and wellness of minority communities. In some cases, this has led to community organizing and social activism, which has been central to EJ since its inception.

9.4 Taking Action

EJ is not simply an academic field; it is also a social movement for change. The Environmental Justice Movement (EJM) combines Civil Rights Movement concerns about inequality and racism with the Environmental Movement of the 1950s and 1960s (Bryant and Hockman 2005; Cole and Foster 2009). The EJM is largely comprised of grassroots organizations whose members belong to aggrieved parties facing environmental injustices that are occurring within their communities, and who are often working class, impoverished, and from minority backgrounds (Cable et al. 2005). These organizations seek to instill in their members the self-determination and power that groups and communities need in order to obtain access to resources, fairness, and justice (Agyeman et al. 2016). The EJM is not primarily concerned with achieving an equitable societal distribution of environmental risks and benefits; instead, the movement focuses on pursuing safe, healthy, and equitable living environments for all, in the present as well as in the future, through clean jobs, a sustainable economy, affordable housing, and social justice for diverse people (Cole and Foster 2009).

Many trace the start of the EJM to 1982 in Warren County, NC. This case involved distributional injustice wherein the predominantly black community of Afton was targeted with a landfill for polychlorinated biphenyl (PCB)-contaminated soil (created through illegal dumping) that threatened the health and quality of life for surrounding communities (Agyeman et al. 2016; Pulido 2017; Bryant and Hockman 2005). The aggrieved residents of Warren County, NC mobilized and protested the siting of the landfill, with support from key political and religious figures. The landfill was created in Warren County despite the strong resistance. Consequently, the US federal government requested an analysis of the correlation between the siting of toxic waste facilities and the racial and sociodemographic makeup of surrounding communities (GAO 1983). Findings from this analysis of Warren County and three additional communities containing hazardous waste landfills showed that there were higher levels of black and low-income residents living in the same zip codes as the toxic dump sites. This study fueled the development of the EJM and subsequent distributive EJ research.

Since the EJM's inception, the movement has enhanced the definition of environment to include where people live, work, eat, play, and pray (as opposed to being limited to wilderness preservation) while prioritizing the environmental concerns of predominantly urban, poor, and racial/ethnic minority communities (Sicotte and Brulle 2017; Agyeman et al. 2016). The EJM has evolved since its initial focus on stopping the proliferation of incinerators and landfills. Today, the EJM includes various areas of concern like air pollution, clean water, food justice, Indigenous rights, energy justice, just sustainability, climate justice, as well as place-making and sense of community (Agyeman et al. 2016; Sicotte and Brulle 2017; Pellow 2017). This expansion is reflected in the USEPA's (2019) current definition of EJ:

> Environmental justice is the fair treatment and meaningful involvement of all people regardless of race, color, national origin, or income, with respect to the development, implementation, and enforcement of environmental laws, regulations, and policies. This goal will be achieved when everyone enjoys the same degree of protection from environmental and health hazards, and equal access to the decision-making process to have a healthy environment in which to live, learn, and work.

The reach of the EJM has spread from local and US national scales to global scales (Agyeman et al. 2016). Leaders of the EJM have united across the globe as a result of economic globalization and transnational movement of industrial pollution from the Global North to the Global South (Pellow and Brulle 2005; Brulle and Pellow 2005a, b). Also, global expansion of the EJM has involved the inclusion of social movement leaders in international conferences where they have been able to connect environmental struggles at the local scale to those of other people undergoing environmental injustice at the global scale (Bryant and Hockman 2005). Though international progress has been made by governing bodies and influential EJM organizations, there is still more work to be done in terms of increasing civil society's access to international environmental decision-making (Ciplet et al. 2015; Sicotte and Brulle 2017; Brulle and Essoka 2005).

9.4.1 Policy and Legislative Action

Central to the EJM is the demand for equal decision-making opportunities for all communities (Bell and Carrick 2017; Schlosberg 2009). As we have discussed, procedural injustices tied to the lack of political influence can often lead to significant environmental injustices and poor health outcomes for marginalized communities. This can be corrected by recognizing and including marginalized people in decision-making that affects their health, communities, and livelihoods (Bell and Carrick 2017). In this context, procedural environmental justice involves marginalized populations "speaking for [themselves]," having a "seat at the table," and demanding "equal, informed, respectful participation" in all environmental decision-making (Schlosberg 2009, p. 66; Bell and Carrick 2017; Cole and Foster 2009; Bryant and Hockman 2005).

The EJM has also pressured the federal government to create equitable environmental legislature. In 1986, for example, the Reagan administration passed the Emergency Planning and Community Right-to-Know Act (EPCRA). This requires industries to report on the storage, use, and release of hazardous chemicals to all levels of government, mainly in efforts to increase public health and access to critical information in times of emergency (USEPA 2017). The Clinton administration implemented the Executive Order (EO) 12898 in 1994 to encourage federal agencies to consider their disparate environmental impacts on minority and low-income communities. While this serves as an important moment in the EJM, it nonetheless exists as a recommended responsibility rather than a policy remedy; that is to say, there are no mechanisms inherent to EO 12898 that can facilitate the resolution of environmental injustices (Abel and Stephan 2017; Gordon and Harley 2005). Hundreds of complaints relating to disparate environmental impacts of federal actions are filed each year, but none have been successfully acted upon due to the lack of any binding requirements associated with EO 12898 (Foster 2017; Gordon and Harley 2005).

US federal priorities to achieve EJ are highly sensitive to administrative changes. During the Obama administration, EJ issues dramatically rose in importance within the EPA. This was influenced by Lisa Jackson's appointment as EPA Administrator under President Obama. As the first female, black person ever appointed as EPA Administrator, Jackson advocated for legislation to limit carbon emissions and greenhouse gases, thereby attempting to address major sources of contemporary environmental inequities (Nealy 2009). During her term, the EPA itself aimed to integrate EJ into its political programs through efforts Plan EJ 2014, Plan EJ 2020, and various EPA funding grants; it also created environmental policy for federally recognized Indigenous tribes, an EJ screening and mapping tool for statistical and spatial analysis, and two guidance documents for regulatory actions (Abel and Stephan 2017). Many of those steps forward have been undone by the Trump administration, which, since 2017, has sought to deregulate polluting industries and increase fossil fuel production (Pulido et al. 2019). This transition has the potential to deepen US environmental injustices. As such, it is important for the EJM to continue advocating for procedural justice and thereby challenge the current administration.

9.5 Conclusion

In summary, environmental benefits and risks are inequitably distributed throughout our societies. Social position—including race, ethnicity, socioeconomic status, gender, and other aspects of identity—greatly influences the degree to which people are exposed to environmental hazards. When hazards become disproportionately concentrated in marginalized communities, it constitutes environmental injustice. Environmental injustices typically degrade the health and opportunities of those affected, reinforcing the marginalization that they experience. In no place is this pattern of environmental injustice better documented than the United States, where ample evidence indicates that racial and ethnic minorities, people of low socioeconomic status, immigrants, and other underrepresented communities have been inequitably environmentally burdened. As the scope of environmental justice research and practice has expanded, similar disparities have been discovered in Europe, Latin America, and Asia, among other world regions. Thus, the social processes and structures responsible for environmental injustices, such as institutional racism, green crime, and the prioritization of capital above human welfare, are by no means limited to the United States.

Within this context, the pursuit of environmental justice research is of utmost importance. All people, regardless of their social positioning, are entitled to safe environments, economic opportunities, and equitable access to the decision-making processes that affect their communities. Ongoing innovation in environmental justice research has the potential to inform social action to address environmental injustices on the ground. In the United States, for example, social actions to address environmental injustice should recognize recent findings that have documented environmental inequities within broad racial-ethnic groups (e.g., for foreign-born Hispanic Americans), and environmental injustices faced by previously ignored groups (e.g., Asian Americans, same-sex partners, or people with disabilities). Such advances could help inform new policies that are more specifically attuned to the varied injustices that affect diverse communities. In the near term, environmental justice analysts should examine how the Trump administration's environmentally- and socially-unconscionable actions have influenced environmental injustices in United States. The new field of green crime may provide particularly useful perspectives for such analyses.

To foster a global perspective, it will be important to expand the focus of environmental justice to additional world regions. While studies have been advanced in Latin America, Europe, and Asia, the global body of knowledge remains limited when compared to the United States. The underdevelopment of environmental justice research worldwide may stymie the creation of equitable, regionally-specific policies that could more effectively redress environmental injustices (Foster 2017; Abel 2008; O'Neill 2000). Developing regionally-specific policies that focus on the needs of particular communities, coupled with mechanisms to incentivize environmental responsibility on behalf of corporations and states, might serve to promote environmental justice across the world. Given the current state of environmental governance, achieving environmental justice will necessitate deeper integration of research with political advocacy.

References

Abel, T., & Stephan, M. (2017). Streams of toxic and hazardous waste disparities, politics, and policy. In R. Holifield, J. Chakraborty, & G. Walker (Eds.), *The Routledge handbook of environmental justice* (pp. 25–36, 311–326). New York, NY: Routledge.

Abel, T. D. (2008). Skewed riskscapes and environmental injustice: A case study of metropolitan St. Louis. *Environmental Management, 42*(2), 232–248.

Agyeman, J., Schlosberg, D., Craven, L., & Matthews, C. (2016). Trends and directions in environmental justice: From inequality to everyday life, community and just sustainabilities. *Annual Review of Environment and Resources, 41,* 321–340.

Aldinger, P. E. (2013). Addressing environmental justice concerns in developing countries: Mining in Nigeria, Uganda and Ghana. *Georgetown International Environmental Law Review, 26,* 345.

Ard, K. (2015). Trends in exposure to industrial air toxins for different racial and socioeconomic groups: A spatial and temporal examination of environmental inequality in the US from 1995 to 2004. *Social Science Research, 53*, 375–390.

Ash, M., & Boyce, J. K. (2018). Racial disparities in pollution exposure and employment at US industrial facilities. *Proceedings of the National Academy of Sciences, 115*(42), 10636–10641.

Basu, P., & Chakraborty, J. (2016). Environmental justice implications of industrial hazardous waste generation in India: A national scale analysis. *Environmental Research Letters, 11*(12), 125001.

Bell, D., & Carrick, J. (2017). Procedural environmental justice. In R. Holifield, J. Chakraborty, & G. Walker (Eds.), *The Routledge handbook of environmental justice* (pp. 25–36, 101–112). New York, NY: Routledge.

Bonds, E. (2016). Legitimating the environmental injustices of war: Toxic exposures and media silence in Iraq and Afghanistan. *Environmental Politics, 25*(3), 395–413.

Brindal, E. (2007). Asia-Pacific: Justice for climate refugees. *Alternative Law Journal, 32*(4), 240–241.

Brulle, R., & Essoka, J. (2005). Whose environmental justice? An analysis of the governance structure of environmental justice organizations in the United States. In D. Pellow & R. Brulle (Eds.), *Power, justice, and the environment: A critical appraisal of the environmental justice movement* (pp. 205–218). Cambridge, MA: MIT Press.

Brulle, R., & Pellow, D. (2005a). Environmental justice: Human health and environmental inequalities. *Annual Review of Public Health, 27*(1), 103–124.

Brulle, R., & Pellow, D. (2005b). The future of environmental justice movements. In D. Pellow & R. Brulle (Eds.), *Power, justice, and the environment: A critical appraisal of the environmental justice movement* (pp. 293–300). Cambridge, MA: MIT Press.

Bryant, B. (Ed.). (1995). *Environmental justice: Issues, policies, and solutions*. Washington, DC: Island Press.

Bryant, B., & Hockman, E. (2005). A brief comparison of the civil rights movement and the environmental justice movement. In D. Pellow & R. Brulle (Eds.), *Power, justice, and the environment: A critical appraisal of the environmental justice movement* (pp. 23–36). Cambridge, MA: MIT Press.

Bullard, R. (1993). Race and environmental justice in the United States. *Yale Journal of International Law,* 319–335.

Bullard, R. (1994). *Dumping in Dixie: Race, class, and environmental quality* (2nd ed.). Boulder, CO: Westview Press.
Bullard, R., & Johnson, G. (2000). Environmentalism and public policy: Environmental justice: Grassroots activism and its impact on public policy decision making. *Journal of Social Issues, 56*(3), 555–578.
Bullard, R., & Lewis, J. (1996). *Environmental justice and communities of color.* San Francisco, CA: Sierra Club Books.
Cable, S., Mix, T., & Hastings, D. (2005). Mission impossible? Environmental justice activists' collaborations with professional environmentalists and with academics. In D. Pellow & R. Brulle (Eds.), *Power, justice, and the environment: A critical appraisal of the environmental justice movement* (pp. 55–90). Cambridge, MA: MIT Press.
Casey, J. A., Morello-Frosch, R., Mennitt, D., Fristrup, K., Ogburn, E., & James, P. (2017). Race/ethnicity, socioeconomic status, residential segregation, and spatial variation in noise exposure in the contiguous United States. *Environmental Health Perspectives, 125*(7), 077017.
Cha, J. (2006). Environmental justice in rural South Asia: Applying lessons learned from the united states in fighting for indigenous communities' rights and access to common resources. *Georgetown International Environmental Law Review, 19,* 185–207.
Chakraborty, J. (2009). Automobiles, air toxics, and adverse health risks: Environmental inequities in Tampa Bay, Florida. *Annals of the Association of American Geographers, 99*(4), 674–697.
Chakraborty, J., & Basu, P. (2019). Linking industrial hazards and social inequalities: Environmental injustice in Gujarat, India. *International Journal of Environmental Research and Public Health, 16*(1), 42.
Chakraborty, J., Collins, T., & Grineski, S. (2017). Cancer risks from exposure to vehicular air pollution: A household level analysis of intra-ethnic heterogeneity in Miami. *Florida. Urban Geography, 38*(1), 112–136.
Chakraborty, J., & Green, D. (2014). Australia's first national level quantitative environmental justice assessment of industrial air pollution. *Environmental Research Letters, 9*(4), 044010.
Ciplet, D., J. Roberts, T., & Mizan R. (2015). *Power in a warming world: The new global politics of climate change and the remaking of environmental inequality.* Cambridge, MA: MIT Press.
Cole, L. W., & Foster, S. R. (2009). *From the ground up: Environmental racism and the environmental justice movement.* New York, NY: New York University Press.
Collins, T., Grineski, S., Chakraborty, J., & McDonald, Y. (2011). Understanding environmental health inequalities through comparative intracategorical analysis: Racial/ethnic disparities in cancer risks from air toxics in El Paso County, Texas. *Health and Place, 17*(1), 335–344.
Collins, T., Grineski, S., & Morales, D. (2017a). Environmental injustice and sexual minority health disparities: A national study of inequitable health risks from air pollution among same-sex partners. *Social Science and Medicine, 191,* 38–47.
Collins, T., Grineski, S., & Morales, D. (2017b). Sexual orientation, gender, and environmental injustice: Unequal carcinogenic air pollution risks in greater Houston. *Annals of the American Association of Geographers, 107*(1), 72–92.
Commission for Racial Justice United Church of Christ. (1987). *Toxic wastes and race in the United States: A national report on the racial and socio-economic characteristics of communities with hazardous waste sites.* New York, NY: United Church of Christ Commission for Racial Justice.
Cunningham, S., Ruben, J., & Venkat Narayan, K. (2008). Health of foreign-born people in the United States: A review. *Health and Place, 14*(4), 623–635.
Cutter, S. (1995). Race, class and environmental justice. *Progress in Human Geography, 19*(1), 111–122.
Downey, L., & Hawkins, B. (2008). Single-mother families and air pollution. *Social Science Quarterly, 89*(2), 523–536.
Evans, G., & Kantrowitz, E. (2002). Socioeconomic status and health: The potential role of environmental risk exposure. *Annual Review of Public Health, 23*(1), 303–331.
Fan, X., Lam, K. C., & Yu, Q. (2012). Differential exposure of the urban population to vehicular air pollution in Hong Kong. *Science of the Total Environment, 426,* 211–219.

Foster, S. (2017). Vulnerability, equality and environmental justice: The potential and limits of law. In R. Holifield, J. Chakraborty, & G. Walker, G. (Eds.), *The Routledge handbook of environmental justice* (pp. 136–148). New York, NY: Routledge.

Fundacion Terram. (2014). *Balance Ambiental 2014. Sacrificando Chile Por la Inversion.* Presidenta: Zonas de sacrifico o justiciar ambiental?, Santiago, www.terram.ck/wpcontent/uploads/2015/01/BALANCE_AMBIENTAL_TERRAM_2014.pdf.

Gochfeld, M., & Burger, J. (2011). Disproportionate exposures in environmental justice and other populations: The importance of outliers. *American Journal of Public Health, 101*(SUPPL. 1), 53–64.

Gordon, H., & Harley, K. (2005). Environmental justice and the legal system. In D. N. Pellow & R. J. Brulle (Eds.), *Power, justice, and the environment: A critical appraisal of the environmental justice movement* (pp. 153–170). Cambridge, MA: MIT Press.

Gouldson, A. (2006). Do firms adopt lower standards in poorer areas? Corporate social responsibility and environmental justice in the EU and the US. *Area, 38*(4), 402–412.

Government Accounting Office (GAO). (1983). *Siting of hazardous waste landfills and their correlation with racial and economic status of surrounding communities*. GAO/RCED-83-168.

Gray, S. C., Edwards, S. E., & Lynn, M. (2013). Race, socioeconomic status, and air pollution exposure in North Carolina. *Environmental Research, 126,* 152–158.

Grineski, S., & Collins, T. (2010). Environmental injustices in transnational context: Urbanization and industrial hazards in El Paso/Ciudad Juárez. *Environment and Planning A, 42*(6), 1308–1327.

Grineski, S., Collins, T., & Chakraborty, J. (2013). Hispanic heterogeneity and environmental injustice: Intra-ethnic patterns of exposure to cancer risks from traffic-related air pollution in Miami. *Population and Environment, 35*(1), 26–44.

Grineski, S., Collins, T., McDonald, Y., Aldouri, R., Aboargob, F., Eldeb, A. … Velázquez-Angulo, G. (2015). Double exposure and the climate gap: changing demographics and extreme heat in Ciudad Juárez, Mexico. *Local Environment, 20*(2), 180–201.

Grineski, S., Collins, T., & Morales, D. (2017). Asian Americans and disproportionate exposure to carcinogenic hazardous air pollutants: A national study. *Social Science and Medicine, 185,* 71–80.

Grineski, S., & Juárez-Carrillo, P. (2012). Environmental injustice in the US-Mexico border region. In *Social justice in the US-Mexico border region* (pp. 179–198). Dordrecht, The Netherlands: Springer.

Harlan, S., Brazel, A., Prashad, L., Stefanov, W., & Larsen, L. (2006). Neighborhood microclimates and vulnerability to heat stress. *Social Science and Medicine, 63*(11), 2847–2863.

Harper, K., Steger, T., & Filčák, R. (2009). Environmental justice and Roma communities in Central and Eastern Europe. *Environmental Policy and Governance, 19*(4), 251–268.

Harris, S., & Harper, B. (1997). A native American exposure scenario. *Risk Analysis, 17*(6), 789–795.

Harris, S., & Harper, B. (2011). A method for tribal environmental justice analysis. *Environmental Justice, 4*(4), 231–237.

Hernandez, M., Collins, T., & Grineski, S. (2015). Immigration, mobility, and environmental injustice: A comparative study of Hispanic people's residential decision-making and exposure to hazardous air pollutants in Greater Houston, Texas. *Geoforum, 60,* 83–94.

Hunter, L. (2006). The spatial association between U.S. immigrant residential concentration and environmental hazards. *International Migration Review, 34*(2), 460.

Jenerette, G., Harlan, S., Brazel, A., Jones, N., Larsen, L., & Stefanov, W. (2007). Regional relationships between surface temperature, vegetation, and human settlement in a rapidly urbanizing ecosystem. *Landscape Ecology, 22*(3), 353–365.

Jiménez, J. (2015). *Desigualdad, concentración del ingreso y tributación sobre las altas rentas en América Latina*. CEPAL.

Jones, A., Brainard, J., Bateman, I., & Lovett, A. (2009). Equity of access to public parks in Birmingham, England. *Environmental Research Journal, 3*(2), 237–256.

Laurent, E. (2011). Issues in environmental justice within the European Union. *Ecological Economics, 70*(11), 1846–1853.

Laurian, L. (2008). Environmental injustice in France. *Journal of Environmental Planning and Management, 51*(1), 55–79.

Leonard, L. (2018). Mining corporations, democratic meddling, and environmental justice in South Africa. *Social Sciences, 7*(12), 259.

Lersch, K., & Hart, T. (2014). Environmental justice, lead, and crime: Exploring the spatial distribution and impact of industrial facilities in Hillsborough County, Florida. *Sociological Spectrum, 34*(1), 1–21.

Liévanos, R. (2015). Race, deprivation, and immigrant isolation: The spatial demography of air-toxic clusters in the continental United States. *Social Science Research, 54,* 50–67.

Liu, L. (2010). Made in China: Cancer villages. *Environment: Science and Policy for Sustainable Development, 52*(2), 8–21.

Lynch, M. (1990). The greening of criminology: A perspective for the 1990's. *The Critical Criminologist, 2*(3), 3–4, 11–12.

Lynch, M., & Barrett, K. (2018). Environmental crime and justice: A green criminological examination. In R. Holifield, J. Chakraborty, & G. Walker (Eds.), *The Routledge handbook of environmental justice* (pp. 425–436). New York, NY: Routledge.

Lynch, M., & Stretesky, P. (2013). Green criminology in the United States. In P. Beirne & N. South (Eds.), *Issues in green criminology* (pp. 248–291). Oregon, WA: Willan.

Lynch, M., & Stretesky, P. (2014). *Exploring green criminology*. London: Routledge.

Maloney, M. (2014). Environmental justice network australia-where to from here. *Asia Pacific Journal of Environmental Law, 17,* 155–162.

Massey, D. (1985). Ethnic residential segregation: A theoretical synthesis and empirical review. *Sociology and Social Research, 69*(3), 315–350.

McCall, L. (2005). The complexity of intersectionality. *Signs, 30,* 1771–1800.

Middleton, C. (2012). Transborder environmental justice in regional energy trade in mainland South-East Asia. *ASEAS-Österreichische Zeitschrift für Südostasienwissenschaften, 5*(2), 292–315.

Mohai, P., Pellow, D., & Roberts, T. J. (2009). Environmental justice. *Annual Review of Environment and Resources, 405,* 405–430.

Nealy, M. (2009). 'Green' for all. *Diverse Issues in Higher Education, 26*(13), 7–9.

Omer, I., & Or, U. (2005). Distributive environmental justice in the city: Differential access in two mixed Israeli cities. *Tijdschrift voor economische en sociale geografie, 96*(4), 433–443.

O'Neill, C. A. (2000). Variable justice: Environmental standards, contaminated fish, and acceptable risk to Native peoples. *Stanford Environmental Law Journal, 19,* 3–120.

Pais, J., Crowder, K., & Downey, L. (2014). Unequal trajectories: Racial and class differences: In residential exposure to industrial hazard. *Social Forces, 92*(3), 1189–1215.

Pellow, D. (2000). Environmental inequality formation: Toward a theory of environmental injustice. *American Behavioral Scientist, 43*(4), 581–601.

Pellow, D. (2007). *Resisting global toxics: Transnational movements for environmental justice*. Cambridge, MA: MIT Press.

Pellow, D. (2017). Environmental justice movements and political opportunity structures. In R. Holifield, J. Chakraborty, & G. Walker (Eds.), *The Routledge handbook of environmental justice* (pp. 37–49). New York, NY: Routledge.

Pellow, D., & Brulle, R. (2005). Power, justice, and the environment: Toward critical environmental justice studies. In D. Pellow & R. Brulle (Eds.), *Power, justice, and the environment: A critical appraisal of the environmental justice movement* (pp. 1–22). Cambridge, MA: MIT Press.

Perrotta, D. (2016). Processing tomatoes in the era of the retailing revolution: Mechanization and migrant labour in northern and southern Italy. In *Migration and agriculture* (pp. 82–100). New York, NY: Routledge.

Pulido, L. (2015). Geographies of race and ethnicity 1: White supremacy vs white privilege in environmental racism research. *Progress in Human Geography, 39*(6), 809–817.

Pulido, L. (2017). Historicizing the personal and the political: Evolving racial formations and the environmental justice movement. In R. Holifield, J. Chakraborty, & G. Walker (Eds.), *The Routledge handbook of environmental justice* (pp. 15–24). New York, NY: Routledge.

Pulido, L., Bruno, T., Faiver-Serna, C., & Galentine, C. (2019). Environmental deregulation, spectacular racism, and White Nationalism in the Trump Era. *Annals of the American Association of Geographers, 109*(2), 520–532.

Quach, T., Liu, R., Nelson, D. O., Hurley, S., Von Behren, J., Hertz, A., et al. (2014). Disaggregating data on Asian American and Pacific Islander women to provide new insights on potential exposures to hazardous air pollutants in California. *Cancer Epidemiology, Biomarkers & Prevention, 23*(11), 2218–2228.

Raddatz, L., & Mennis, J. (2013). Environmental justice in Hamburg, Germany. *The Professional Geographer, 65*(3), 495–511.

Ruggiero, V., & South, N. (2010). Green criminology and dirty collar crime. *Critical Criminology, 18*(4), 251–262.

Schlosberg, D. (2009). *Defining environmental justice: Theories, movements, and nature*. Oxford: Oxford University Press.

Shmueli, D. (2008). Environmental justice in the Israeli context. *Environment and Planning A, 40* (10), 2384–2401.

Sicotte, D., & Brulle, R. (2017). Social movements for environmental justice through the lens of social movement theory. In R. Holifield, J. Chakraborty, & G. Walker (Eds.), *The Routledge handbook of environmental justice* (pp. 25–36). New York, NY: Routledge.

Spring, A. (2013). Declining segregation of same-sex partners: Evidence from Census 2000 and 2010. *Population Research and Policy Review, 32*(5), 687–716.

Stretesky, P. (2003). The distribution of air lead levels across U.S. Counties: Implications for the production of racial inequality. *Sociological Spectrum, 23*(1), 91–118.

Stretesky, P., Long, M., & Lynch, M. (2013). The treadmill of crime: Political economy and green criminology. New York, NY: Routledge.

Steger, T., & Filcak, R. (2008). Articulating the basis for promoting environmental justice in Central and Eastern Europe. *Environmental Justice, 1*(1), 49–53.

Tal, A. (2002). *Pollution in a promised land: An environmental history of Israel*. Berkeley, CA: University of California Press.

Temper, L., del Bene, D., & Martinez-Alier, J. (2015). Mapping the frontiers and front lines of global environmental justice: The EJAtlas. *Journal of Political Ecology, 22,* 255–278.

United Nations. (2014). *World urbanization prospect 2014: Highlights*. United Nations Publications. www.compassion.com/multimedia/world-urbanization-prospects.pdf.

USEPA Office of Land and Emergency Management. (2017). *The emergency planning and community right-to-know act fact sheet*. https://www.epa.gov/sites/production/files/2017-08/documents/epcra_fact_sheet_overview_8-2-17.pdf.

USEPA. (2019). *Environmental justice*. https://www.epa.gov/environmentaljustice.

Vasquez, A., Lukas, M., Salgado, M., & Mayonga, J. (2018). Urban environmental (in)justice in Latin America: The case of Chile. In R. Holifield, J. Chakraborty, & G. Walker (Eds.), *The Routledge handbook of environmental justice* (pp. 556–566). New York, NY: Routledge.

Webster, P. (2005). *White dust black death: The tragedy of asbestos mining at Baryulgil*. Trafford Publishing.

FSC
www.fsc.org
MIX
Papier | Fördert
gute Waldnutzung
FSC® C083411

Kolibri 360 GmbH
Ferdinand-Jühlke-Straße 7
99095 Erfurt, Deutschland
produktsicherheit@kolibri360.de